How To Be Awake

(So You Can Sleep Through the Night)

Heather
Darwall-Smith

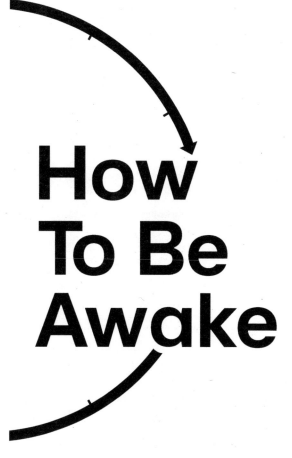

How
To Be
Awake

(So You Can Sleep
Through the Night)

Thorsons

Thorsons
An imprint of HarperCollins*Publishers*
1 London Bridge Street
London SE1 9GF

www.harpercollins.co.uk

HarperCollins*Publishers*
Macken House, 39/40 Mayor Street Upper
Dublin 1, D01 C9W8, Ireland

First published by Thorsons 2025

1 3 5 7 9 10 8 6 4 2

A catalogue record of this book is available from the British Library

ISBN 978-0-00-866655-2

Printed and bound in the UK using 100% renewable electricity at CPI Group (UK) Ltd

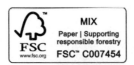

Contents

Introduction

Let's start with an idea that might challenge you: not sleeping perfectly isn't a catastrophe. Humans have lived with restless nights, wakeful hours and uneven sleep patterns for centuries. Our bodies are resilient; if we can get our minds out of the way, our bodies know how to recover. But somewhere along the line the story around sleep became distorted. We're told that without a flawless eight hours, we're failing – that if we don't optimise every hour of our existence, we're at risk of becoming unhealthy, unproductive and unhappy. In a world that never sleeps, many of us have forgotten how to rest, let alone sleep. Your bed has become something to fear.

Chasing sleep: why trying harder can keep you awake

The more we obsess over 'optimising' every detail of our night – to perfect it, measure it, fix it – the more anxious and awake we've become. Maybe you know this feeling all too well. You've tried the routines, the supplements, the apps, hoping to finally conquer sleep. But if you're here, perhaps you've realised that sleep doesn't respond to fear or control. So here's the paradox: the harder you chase sleep, the further it runs away.

Many people seek to address their sleep issues by paying intense attention to what happens just before they go to bed, and at night. This is entirely understandable, but it's not often effective. This book shifts the focus to your entire 24-hour rhythm, helping you see how your waking life shapes your nights – an often-overlooked perspective. It encourages you to embrace acceptance and self-compassion, freeing you from the burden of rigid sleep expectations. While many books prescribe universal solutions, this one prioritises flexibility, offering you tools and insights to experiment with, so you can discover what truly works for your unique needs, without the pressure of a 'one-size-fits-all' approach.

Flip the script: your nights follow your days

If you're struggling with chronic sleep issues, looking deeper and exploring what else might be at play is essential. Often, what's needed is a combination of clarity – what's really going on in terms of your support systems and stress management – and a return to simple pleasures that reconnect you to yourself. Medical issues aside (and I'll come on to those), real rest comes from living your life in a way that invites sleep naturally and effortlessly, without force or struggle.

Maybe this sounds familiar: it's 3 a.m., and you're lying awake, staring at the ceiling. Anxiety creeps in as the minutes tick by. You've tried everything – turning off screens, practising breathing exercises, sipping valerian tea – but sleep remains elusive. Your mind races with thoughts of the exhausting day ahead, filled with meetings, deadlines and the fear of making mistakes. By morning, you drag yourself out of bed, already dreading another sleepless night. The cycle continues and you simply don't know what to do.

I can't give you a formula for 'perfect' sleep. There is no quick fix, no magic ritual. More than that, there are sometimes structural issues in place like a lack of sound-proofing in your home or a shift-pattern that moves all over the place, but do not despair. In this book, we're going to flip the script and focus on how you live during the day so that sleep can follow at night.

As an accredited UKCP psychotherapist specialising in sleep, I work with those who are exhausted by sleepless nights, anxious thoughts and restless minds. I'm professionally bound to maintain confidentiality. The people and scenarios you'll encounter in this book are fictional. To the hundreds of individuals I've worked with – both in private practice and in sleep clinics – your stories are safe with me. Yet, many of the challenges around sleep are universal and you may recognise pieces of your own journey here.

Sleep fascinates me. Biologically, we're all wired to sleep. And yet, for so many, it becomes a battleground. In many ways, it's not a surprise. We live in a world that pulls us out of rhythm, where we light up the night, push our limits and rarely slow down. The pandemic disrupted our lives, routines and sense of security. It left many of us in a perpetual state of alert, and some of us still struggle to feel safe enough to rest.

Our bodies are deeply rhythmic, operating on an internal clock known as the circadian rhythm. This clock not only responds to environmental cues, such as light and darkness, but also anticipates and regulates virtually all of our bodily functions, most notably the sleep–wake cycle. But stress, irregular routines and constant screen exposure can throw that rhythm out of balance, leaving us out of sync. When brain chemicals like serotonin and melatonin fall out of alignment and cortisol – the stress hormone – takes over, our bodies can't find rest. Instead, we're left in constant churn, unable to switch off.

Our culture often sacrifices sleep on the altar of productivity. In his book, *The Secret Pulse of Time: Making Sense of Life's Scarcest Commodity*, journalist Stefan Klein observes that, 'time is life's scarcest commodity.'[1] And he's right – we're constantly told to optimise every minute. But without sleep, we're neither productive nor truly well. Sleep isn't something we can fully control or perfect; it's personal, fluid and different for everyone. Instead of prescribing rigid routines, this book invites you to approach sleep with curiosity. It's about exploring what genuinely works for *you*, rather than chasing the latest trend or one-size-fits-all advice.

The maths of modern life: where does the time go?

This reality of why sleep goes wrong becomes more apparent when you break down your daily demands. If you don't actively protect your time for sleep and rest, they'll be the first things to go. A viral social media post from a recent college graduate illustrated this perfectly.[2] They described the exhaustion of the 9-to-5 grind, the financial strain of city living, long commutes and the crushing realisation that their evenings left no room for hobbies, social life, or even rest. Their question summed up what many are feeling: 'How do you have time for a life?'

Let's look at the numbers: there are 24 hours in a day. Subtract 7–9 hours for sleep (we'll address the 8-hour myth in Chapter Two), 8 hours for work, 2 for meals, 2 for personal care and 1–2 hours for commuting. The maths is straightforward: 8 (sleep) + 8 (work) + 2 (meals) + 2 (personal care) + 2 (commute) = 22. That leaves just 2 hours for everything else. And that's before you factor in chores, exercise, children, family time or personal interests. Where's the space for joy, creativity or even boredom? What is going to get squeezed?

This highlights a deeper issue: our collective undervaluing of sleep and rest. For many, sleep is the first thing to be sacrificed in the pursuit of productivity, often for reasons outside our control, whether it's demanding jobs, caregiving responsibilities or economic pressures. By treating sleep as a luxury rather than a necessity, we risk undermining the very things we're trying to protect: our health, our wellbeing and our sanity.

This mindset has deep historical roots. The industrial age brought a focus on efficiency, productivity and maximising output. Time became something to be measured and optimised, leading to the belief that 'time is money'. Sleep, which doesn't deliver immediate results, was pushed aside. But this mentality is out of step with our natural rhythms, and the consequences are becoming harder to ignore.

To sleep well, we need to reframe how we think about time – not as a commodity to be hoarded and spent, but as something that should include and prioritise rest. This includes understanding the importance of sleep, taking breaks during the day and allowing time for recovery after physical exertion. Only then can we start living in a way that genuinely supports our wellbeing. But this isn't just a personal issue. We all need to think about it as private citizens, employers, politicians and policymakers.

Think of tackling sleep issues like solving a Rubik's Cube, where each side represents a different factor: mental health, lifestyle habits, physical conditions, environmental influences and, perhaps most importantly, a sense of safety. Working on one side impacts the others, creating a ripple effect. Adjusting your daily routines and managing stress can often make subtle shifts, supporting better sleep and overall wellbeing.

This book invites you to approach sleep with curiosity, compassion and a willingness to embrace the messy, unpredictable nature of rest. Because most of the time the key to good sleep isn't about trying harder – it's about letting go.

Your body knows how to sleep

Many people rely on medications, and there's no shame in that. In fact, there are situations where medication, when carefully prescribed by a specialist, is not just helpful but absolutely essential. In sleep, however, it is not unusual for them to create a bigger problem. Letting go of the meds can feel terrifying; you might not trust that you can sleep without them. Your fear is valid, and taking things one step at a time is OK. By the end of this book, you'll have a toolbox of strategies to help you find your way to restful sleep. And if one tool doesn't work, try another; flexibility is key.

Sleep isn't something you can control by sheer willpower. Ironically, the harder you try, the more elusive it becomes. This drive for control often stems from a desire for safety, but it can lead to stress and insomnia. Instead of striving to eliminate stress, the goal is to learn how to coexist with it in a healthy way. Just as you can't fully appreciate joy without experiencing frustration, sleep often improves when you acknowledge and accept stress rather than trying to banish it. I don't see stress – as in the fight-or-flight response – as inherently bad. Stress is a life force; it drives you, sharpens you and even protects you. But when stress starts to run the show and becomes chronic, we are in trouble.

When stressed, the mind speeds up – its inner monkey launches into problem-solving mode, speeding up and worrying about the should I, would I, could I's. Lurching between the unknown future and the past that is past, you miss the here and now, yet the here and now is all we have. It's an ironic twist. In a need for control, do you rob yourself of the light-hearted moments that bring genuine happiness and relaxation?

The real challenge isn't eliminating stress but learning how to dial it up or down so you're not always stuck on high alert. Think of developing an internal dimmer switch, not an on/off button. Life isn't about flipping from calm to chaos; it's about modulating and finding the right intensity for each moment. When you master that, stress becomes an ally not an enemy.

Recognise what you can and cannot control. I can't change the fact that it's raining outside, but I can take an umbrella with me when I go out – I can prepare the best I can. Sometimes, even I have a rubbish night of sleep, but I know how to pace myself the next day. Life is full of ups and downs, and we constantly face uncertainty, rapid changes and unexpected turns. And in truth, there are times when losing control is stressful and even frightening, and you will struggle to cope – that is normal.

Similarly, you can't manage global events like economic crises, wars or natural disasters (and doom-scrolling your way through social media isn't going to help). Your nervous system isn't built to handle constant global crises – it's designed to manage what's nearby. So you can learn to gently bring your restless, anxious mind back under control – think of it a bit like coaxing a frightened animal out of a dark corner.

With countless apps and devices promising the perfect night's rest, sleep can start to feel like something we have to 'perform'. This pressure often keeps us awake, fearing we're not measuring up. But sleep is meant to support how we spend our days, not become another measure of productivity or something to get competitive over – who has the best sleep score? Your sleep is unique and can't be compared to others'. It is deeply influenced by genetics, gender, psychology, environment, culture and more. It responds to how we spend our days, and in turn, it shapes how we experience them. A restless night can lead to a sluggish, unproductive day, impacting our mental health and overall wellbeing.

And here's where the relentless push of life comes into play, nudging you, perhaps a bit too roughly, towards an ironic realisation: it might be time to take a breather, to wake up and, quite literally, smell the coffee. The irony of that suggestion in a book about sleep!

When was the last time you paused to savour a cup of coffee, to feel its warmth and enjoy its flavour instead of rushing through it? These little breaks remind us of the good things in life. Instead, invest in the best coffee that you can afford, use the perfect cup and really savour it. It becomes a mindful moment of rest.

So maybe, when you're lying there wide awake at night, all tangled up in the noise of everything you've got going on, take a beat. Stop. Take a few deep breaths – in and out. You might find the calm that's been dodging you in these quiet moments. Ask yourself in the right here, right now, are you safe? What do you need to support yourself? And who knows, as the moments increase from seconds to minutes to hours, that'll be the trick to finally getting some good shuteye.

Throughout this book, I'll share insights and tools to help you build a more relaxed relationship with sleep. For some, that might mean creating a bedtime routine; for others, it could involve addressing deeper psychological issues. Fear of sleeplessness can often be as debilitating as sleeplessness itself. Shifting from anxiety about sleep to acceptance can make all the difference. Always remember – biologically, your body knows how to do this.

Make this book work for you

We're bombarded with advice about supplements, routines and strict schedules, but what works for one person may not work for another. Our journey together will explore these individual variations, offering flexible guidance to help you find what suits your life. It's not about adhering to the latest trend (I see you, sleepy girl mocktail[3]); it's about experimenting with different approaches and discovering what supports your unique needs.

Another significant issue is whether your expectations around sleep are realistic. Advice is everywhere – newspapers, books (yes, I see the irony), podcasts and more. Many of these sources promote elaborate routines and expensive supplements (often backed by lucrative partnerships), as the ultimate path to perfect sleep. Cold showers, strict schedules, intermittent fasting – each presented as a 'must' for restful nights.

But in my work, I see the downside of these rigid, restrictive approaches. You're not a machine and you're not in control of every aspect of your life. Your body constantly changes, and a structured yet flexible approach will serve you far better. Real rest is about working with your body, not forcing it into someone else's formula.

Taking every piece of sleep advice as gospel can lead to a rigid, stressful approach to bedtime. Professor Matthew Walker, author of the groundbreaking book *Why We Sleep*,[4] even admitted on the Huberman Podcast[5] that he may have been 'a little too puritanical'. His book brought the importance of sleep to the forefront, but I've lost count of how many people have told me it left them feeling more anxious than reassured.

For Walker, carefully managing sleep means selecting a gym based on the aspect of its windows to optimise his circadian rhythm – a great approach if you have the luxury to make that choice. But what works for a sleep scientist may not work for a single mother juggling three kids and a full-time job or a night-shift worker whose schedule is beyond their control. Sleep is deeply personal, and what works for one person may not work for another. Some people thrive on seven to nine hours of uninterrupted rest, while others do well with less. Our journey together will explore these individual differences, offering insights and tools to help you discover what works best for you.

I aim to cut through the noise without the pressure of adhering to every latest trend. This book is about engaging your curiosity, looking beyond the noise, and integrating practical tools and ways of thinking into your life in a natural and supportive way rather than being prescriptive and overwhelming. I am not a fan of rigid routines and have repeatedly seen how detrimental they can be – avoiding an unexpected night out because of your sleep routine. Sometimes it's about saying, 'fuck it' and doing it anyway and benefiting from a wild night out with friends. Other times, it's about learning when you need to say no.

If you have insomnia, cognitive behavioural therapy for insomnia (CBT-I) is one of the most effective treatments available, helping about 70–80 per cent of affected people improve their sleep. It typically includes a range of strategies that help you to identify and change unhelpful thoughts about sleep, establish healthy sleep habits, learn relaxation techniques and address anxieties around bedtime. It also doesn't suit everyone. So what about the 20–30 per cent for whom it doesn't work? Often, other factors are at play. Many people with sleep issues face multiple overlapping challenges, from unresolved stress and trauma to coexisting health conditions. This is the territory where I focus my work, through a multi-disciplinary approach.

Sometimes the roots of sleeplessness lie buried in the subconscious, tied to unaddressed grief, unprocessed trauma or an enduring sense that you're not safe. It's not just a matter of counting sheep – it's about the things we carry that keep us alert, even when we're desperate to rest.

Think about it; humans are one of the only species born utterly dependent on others for survival and we're living in a world that feels increasingly chaotic, politically charged and full of rapid, unpredictable change. Even *in utero*, we need others for security. From our first breath we are learning about safety – or the lack of it – in the arms of those who care for us. These early experiences teach us what it means to feel secure, but sadly many of us never experience that safety. Fast-forward to adulthood; many of us exist in a constant state of low-grade alert, stress becoming a normal way of being. Our nervous systems brace for impact, making it nearly impossible to relax fully – let alone sleep deeply.

The nervous system

Your nervous system is the foundation of your survival and well-being, managing both voluntary actions (like moving your hand) and involuntary functions (like breathing). It operates through two key branches: the sympathetic nervous system, which activates your stress response, and the parasympathetic nervous system (PNS), which promotes rest, digestion and sleep. Sleep relies heavily on the parasympathetic system, as it allows your body to relax and enter a state of recovery.

This book will guide you through understanding these systems and how intentional practices, like slowing your breath, can help shift your body into a calm, parasympathetic state, making it easier to fall and stay asleep. Thanks to the brain's incredible adaptability (neuroplasticity), you can train your nervous system to respond more effectively, improving both your sleep quality and overall resilience over time.

If your body's internal alarm is constantly ringing, disrupted sleep isn't a mystery; it's practically a given. Why would you be able to sleep if you aren't safe? – that's dangerous. Take Maria, who came to me frustrated after trying every sleep trick in the book. It wasn't until she began to process the unresolved grief of a past loss that her body finally allowed her to rest. Or Peter, who spent years struggling with insomnia until he faced the childhood trauma that his mind had kept locked away.

And it's not just trauma. Sometimes, other hidden forces are at work – undiagnosed neurodiversity, chronic stress, addiction or physical pain that the body has been holding on to in silence. These are the things that standard sleep advice rarely addresses but that wreak havoc on our ability to unwind.

If this resonates, know you're not alone. We all have these hidden stories and unmet needs that whisper to us in the dark, keeping our minds spinning and our bodies tense. This book invites you to look deeper and explore those layers of experience that may be holding you back from proper rest. Because sometimes, finding sleep isn't about trying harder – it's about understanding what your sleeplessness is trying to tell you and finding a way to rest.

Every individual who prioritises rest and recovery sends out ripples that reach far beyond themselves. And here's the beauty of it all; it sparks a quiet revolution when you take these steps. As more and more people adopt practices that promote restful sleep and a relaxed nervous system, the collective energy of society will begin to shift. It's time to turn the pillow over . . . It's time to rest.

The techniques in this book require an open mind, consistent practice and sustained effort. It may feel ironic, but the responses that disrupt your sleep are often your body's way of trying to protect you – just in ways that don't always serve you well.

People often feel frustrated, saying, 'This doesn't work.' And it's true; sometimes a technique might not work immediately. But that doesn't mean nothing will. Trying something new for the first time at 3 a.m. in a state of panic is unlikely to be effective. Under those conditions, it's no surprise that many approaches fall short.

Think of learning coping skills as building muscle. You don't wait for a crisis to start training; you develop these skills during calm moments, repeating them until they become second nature. By practising when you're at ease, you're building tools that will be there when you need them most. So when stress hits, you'll know what to do – instinctively 'flexing' these new muscles and feeling more grounded and resilient. This proactive approach makes it far less likely you'll abandon these techniques when you need them the most.

Keep a journal

I recommend keeping a journal to record your experiences. When we're sleep-deprived or feeling negative our memories can be unreliable; we often remember things as being worse than they were. Writing things down gives you a clear, objective record of your experiences and helps you 'see' your thoughts more clearly, which can be reassuring during uncertain times.

Adapt to your learning style

Not everyone is a writer, and it's essential to recognise your unique way of processing information. If you learn best by listening, try recording your thoughts on your phone. If you're a visual learner, drawing your ideas or creating diagrams might make things clearer. And if you're hands-on, try using something tactile, like Play-Doh, to explore your thoughts.

- **Immerse yourself**: Dive into the book's ideas about rest and sleep. Sometimes, a single insight can be a game-changer, like finding the correct turn on a Rubik's Cube.
- **Take notes**: Jot down key concepts to help you absorb and remember them.
- **Understand your situation**: Use the tools to assess your sleep patterns and stress levels.
- **Identify triggers**: Recognise the patterns and triggers that may impact your sleep. You can also share this information with your GP for additional support if needed.

Test and learn

Keep it simple; you likely only need a few tools. Don't overcomplicate things. Experiment with different techniques to find what works best for you. Keep track of your progress and note any changes in your sleep patterns or stress levels. This process of testing and refining will help you create a personalised approach to managing stress and improving sleep. Remember – gentle progress is the goal. Practising these techniques during calm periods and planning for more stressful times can significantly improve your ability to handle stress and support better sleep.

Do you have a diagnosable disorder?

When does poor sleep cross the line into a diagnosable disorder? This is a vital question, but it doesn't have a straightforward answer. The distinction often lies in the persistence of the problem, the extent of its impact on your daily life and whether it can be traced to an identifiable cause, such as a physiological or psychological condition. Factors such as genetics, chronotype (our natural sleep patterns), culture and even gender play a role, influencing both our baseline sleep patterns and how we perceive disruptions.

When people think about sleep problems, insomnia is usually the first thing that comes to mind. While insomnia disorder is a clinically recognised condition, it differs significantly from occasional sleeplessness or 'bad' nights of sleep. Insomnia disorder is defined by its persistence (occurring regularly and not tied to a specific situation), its impact (causing significant distress or impairing daily functioning) and its resistance to change despite efforts to improve sleep. Many people self-identify as having insomnia when they're actually experiencing short-term or situational sleep difficulties that don't meet the diagnostic criteria. However it's not always insomnia – there are over 80 diagnosable sleep disorders, each with its own unique causes, symptoms and effects.

Sleep apnea is a common but often undiagnosed condition that occurs when the airway becomes partially or completely blocked during sleep, or when the brain fails to send the signals needed to maintain normal breathing. These disruptions cause fragmented sleep, which can lead to excessive daytime sleepiness and other serious health issues. Many misunderstood sleep problems can be traced back to circadian rhythm disorders – conditions where the internal body clock that regulates your sleep–wake cycle is out of sync with the demands of your environment. Circadian rhythm disorders are not 'bad habits' – they are clinically recognised conditions that involve a disruption in the natural timing of your body's processes. For example, delayed sleep–wake phase disorder (DSWPD) can cause people to struggle with falling asleep until very late at night, while advanced sleep–wake phase disorder (ASWPD) may lead to extreme early morning wakefulness.

As you move through this book, reflect on whether your sleep challenges feel temporary and situational or whether they are persistent, disruptive and resistant to change. Ask yourself: 'Does my sleep problem persist regardless of what I do?' 'Does it affect my ability to function or my quality of life?' If the answer to those questions is 'yes', you may need to see a doctor or specialist. Chapter Seven will delve into recognising when sleep issues may require medical attention and how to seek appropriate help.

Here's a radical thought: perhaps you could enjoy falling asleep!

Imagine that – no longer thinking about sleep with worry! Instead, you might look forward to it. I present the possibility that this is not only achievable but likely. Without anxiety in the way, you can experience the magic that happens as you drift in and out of sleep.

If you experience anxiety about falling asleep, it might seem mind-boggling to think it might be enjoyable and fun. Let's play into the always-on cultural narrative that sleep might be productive! Many studies have shown that one of sleep's most important roles is the consolidation of memory and learning, but there is also another interesting element – a specific neurobiological process known as 'hypnagogia' and the 'hypnagogic state'. This is the dreamy state between wakefulness and sleep where fascinating things happen in your brain. As the parts of your brain that process sensory information – like sights and sounds – begin to quieten down, your thoughts start to blend with the world around you, creating vivid and often surreal experiences. Meanwhile, the default mode network, the brain region responsible for thoughts and memories, becomes more active. This heightened activity fosters new connections, igniting creativity and sparking fresh ideas.

As someone who enjoys the mechanics of how sleep works, I've found that leaning into this state of sleep itself is helpful. Often, when I've been working late into the evening on this book, my mind would be buzzing with complex details. Instead of forcing myself to untangle these thoughts right then and there I've learned to let go, trusting that the hypnagogic state and the sleep that follows will help clarify things overnight. I now see falling asleep as more than just the necessary prelude to a good night's rest – it's an opportunity, a precious moment of mental alchemy where the day's raw materials are turned into something new.

Many artists, inventors and scientists have attributed their breakthrough ideas to this transitional state. For instance, Thomas Edison used to exploit the hypnagogic state intentionally. Edison would hold steel balls in his hands above a metal plate and allow himself to drift off to sleep. As he entered the hypnagogic state, the balls would drop, waking him up, and he would immediately jot down whatever ideas had come to him.[6] While I am not suggesting you go to these places right now, I want to show you that something entirely different is available in the experience of falling asleep or waking up.

Can you think of sleep as a trusted friend? Like any meaningful relationship, it thrives on care and patience. Criticise it or push it away, and it may grow distant. But if you welcome it warmly – creating a safe, inviting space – it will be far more likely to return. Learning how to nurture your connection with sleep can transform it from an elusive guest into a steadfast companion.

CHAPTER ONE

What are we getting wrong about sleep?

For starters, sleep issues aren't always about simple habits like too much caffeine or late-night screen time. Aside from a diagnosable disorder, their roots can be far more complex. Perhaps you don't feel safe or are burdened with a super-busy brain. If so, it might be better to understand sleep problems as a logical response to stress or a world set on a 9-to-5 clock, while your body hasn't got the memo. When your brain and body perceive danger, stress activates the fight-or-flight response – a protective mechanism that keeps you alert, but it will also keep you awake. Awake, you are safe. If your cellular timing (chronotype) says you are a night owl, the 9-to-5 will be hard for you. Recognising these various factors and what is happening for you can change how you approach your sleep issue. It brings space and compassion, opening up the possibility to think differently about what might really be happening.

Sometimes, realising that the problems you are having with sleep are how sleep responds to life opens the door to making changes. You can rest assured that your body is programmed to know how to sleep – but it might have its own ideas about how it does that, ideas that don't fit the 9-to-5 world. Remember, a good night's sleep isn't just about having a nice little routine in the hour before bed; it starts when you wake up.

The science of sleep

Sleep is a natural and recurring state of rest for both the mind and body, essential for health and wellbeing. We haven't evolved out of needing it, so it clearly has an important role. Even in the late 1990s, scientists joked that the main purpose of sleep is 'to cure sleepiness',[1] but we know it does much more and continue to learn all the time. Sleep is an active process involving multiple stages, each with specific functions essential for physical health, memory consolidation and emotional regulation. It's the brain's best friend, providing a space for overnight recovery when the conscious 'you' goes offline. The brain and sleep work in tandem; the brain constantly anticipates and responds to your needs through several biological mechanisms. It works nonstop, 24 hours a day, and sleep allows it to switch to a different mode to recover.

Sleep isn't a static target, and the idea of the 'magic eight hours' is misleading. Sleep is a continually shifting variable, influenced by factors like age, lifestyle and individual needs. Ideally, unless you're a genetic short sleeper,[2] most adults under 60 should be getting between seven to nine hours of sleep each night. As you age, this drops to seven to eight hours a night. The key is to focus less on hitting an exact number and more on understanding and adapting to your body's ever-changing needs. True short sleepers are exceptionally rare, making up less than 1 per cent of the population. Due to specific genetic mutations in genes like DEC2 and ADRB1, they can function perfectly well on just four to six hours of sleep per night. Unlike most people who suffer from lack of sleep, true short sleepers maintain high levels of alertness, productivity and emotional stability. Their unique genetic makeup allows them to get by on significantly less sleep without any adverse consequences.

While it's clear that the longer you are awake the more pressure to sleep will build up, your daily sleep–wake cycles are complex. Research into circadian rhythms – 24-hour cycles regulating bodily functions – shows that every aspect of your physiology follows this daily pattern. If you stay awake all night, you'll feel tired during those hours and wish you were asleep, but come mid-morning of the next day, to your surprise, you have the energy to keep going. You might become exhausted again by mid-afternoon, then, if you haven't slept, dip again in the evening to the point where sleep becomes irresistible. This pattern indicates that your need for sleep increases the longer you stay awake but varies throughout the day.

Understanding sleep as a biological process is incredibly empowering because it reminds us that our bodies are naturally designed for it – sleep is hardwired into our biology. At the core of sleep regulation is a two-process system identified by sleep scientist Alexander Borbély: Process S and Process C. Process S, or 'sleep drive', builds up sleep pressure the longer you're awake, making you feel increasingly tired. Process C, or the 'circadian rhythm', is your internal clock that responds to light and darkness, signalling when to feel alert or drowsy over a 24-hour cycle. Together, these processes determine when you feel sleepy and when you're ready to wake up.[3] Even if you miss out on it, your body doesn't just give up; it compensates through sleep homeostasis – a biological process that regulates your body's need for sleep – prioritising deep, restorative sleep the following night to help you recover. And when you're stressed, your body can adjust your sleep patterns to keep you alert when needed. These mechanisms ensure you get the recovery you need, making sleep your best friend in maintaining health.[4]

Starting to think about sleep as your friend is often a new way of thinking about it. I have seen people tangibly recoil at the thought of it, their relationship with it being so difficult. People with problems with sleep tend to dislike it, hate it, or worse – of all – fear it, which sets off a neurological process that, ironically, makes it even harder to sleep. Why would sleep, your friend, choose to stay with you if it senses you dislike or fear it?

Important – you need to be sleepy to go to sleep!

Two of the most frustrating sleep struggles are lying in bed exhausted but unable to fall asleep, or waking at 3 a.m. and feeling wide awake. Staring at the clock, stressing about lost sleep, only makes it harder to drift off again. The truth is, you can't force sleep if your body isn't ready. The harder you try, the more alert and frustrated you'll feel. Instead, get up and do something relaxing.

If you are not sleepy it's time to do something else. If you reach for your phone, use it intentionally – listen to a guided meditation, calming audiobook or soothing sounds like rain. Avoid email, social media or anything stimulating, and keep notifications off. If your phone isn't appealing, try reading something light, journalling, doodling or doing gentle stretches or yoga. Even small tasks like folding laundry or tidying can help distract your mind.

Even if you don't fall back into a deep sleep or sleep feels light, rest is still valuable. Your body is still recovering, and as we will come to see, staying calm will help build up your biological sleep pressure for the following night, making it more likely you'll get the restorative sleep you need then.

Typically, after 16 to 18 hours of being awake, your body feels ready for sleep. Imagine that, throughout the day, your body is collecting 'sleepiness coins' AKA sleep pressure – a representation of Process S. Each waking hour adds a coin to your stash, and by the time night falls, you need a full 'wallet' of coins to 'buy' a restful night's sleep. If your wallet is light – say, because you've taken a long nap (which uses a few coins) or haven't been awake long enough – it might feel harder to make that purchase.

This build-up is mainly driven by a substance in your brain called adenosine, which accumulates as you stay awake. It serves as a signal, telling your body when it's time to rest. When you sleep, this pressure decreases, as your brain clears adenosine, allowing you to wake up feeling refreshed. However, if you don't get enough sleep, the pressure doesn't fully reset, leading to feelings of tiredness and a stronger urge to sleep – recover – the following night. But if your mind is buzzing with alertness from a stressful day, it can keep you awake, no matter how many coins you've saved. Which is why after a long day at work – filled with back-to-back meetings, endless emails and little movement – it can be tough to fall asleep even if you're physically worn out. It's what people mean when they say they're 'tired but wired'.

The trick to a good night's sleep is not just about collecting enough sleepiness coins – you need to be sleepy to go to sleep – but also timing (Process C) and being ready to sleep. Everyone collects these 'sleep coins' at their own pace. That's why 'morning larks' tend to feel sleepy early in the evening, while 'night owls' often stay alert until much later.

Understanding how sleep pressure and your body's natural rhythms work (Process S and C) can help you better adapt your daily schedule to meet your needs. I've often discussed with people how vital it is to grasp the timing of their biological clock, and we get into that in the next chapter. Some individuals have what's known as a circadian rhythm disorder, where their natural sleep times don't align with conventional schedules. This misalignment makes it essential to wait until you're genuinely sleepy before going to bed. Without that natural alignment between sleepiness and bedtime, you're likely to end up lying awake, feeling frustrated and anxious about not being able to fall asleep.

Understanding whether you have a circadian rhythm disorder can also take a lot of the frustration and emotional toll out of dealing with sleep issues. Many people blame themselves or feel a sense of failure when they struggle to fall asleep at a 'normal' bedtime or wake up on time, thinking it's a matter of willpower or discipline. Knowing that your body's internal clock simply operates on a different schedule can help shift this mindset, reducing self-blame and allowing for a more compassionate, science-based approach to sleep. Instead of forcing yourself into a schedule that doesn't align with your biology, you can focus on strategies that work with your natural rhythms, making sleep feel less like a battle and more like a manageable, achievable goal. This self-understanding can bring a sense of relief and control, helping you approach sleep with less anxiety and more patience.

How to increase sleep pressure – feel sleepy at bedtime

Sleep restriction therapy (SRT) is an evidence-based method to improve sleep quality by increasing sleep pressure (save up sleepiness coins). In clinical comparisons, SRT is often found to be as effective as or more effective than sleep medication for treating chronic insomnia, particularly in the long term. While it may seem counterintuitive – you might think, 'I'm already exhausted, why would I sleep less?' – this approach retrains your brain and body to consolidate and improve sleep naturally. In fact, CBT-I (with SRT as a core component) is recommended as the first-line treatment for insomnia by organisations like the American Academy of Sleep Medicine and the National Institute for Health and Care Excellence (NICE).

When sleep is fragmented and shallow, spending too much time in bed can make it worse. SRT temporarily reduces the time you spend in bed to align with the amount of sleep your body is currently achieving. This boosts **sleep efficiency** (the percentage of time spent asleep, see page 50), increases your natural sleep pressure and promotes deeper, more restorative sleep.

Importantly, the goal is to improve the quality of your sleep through consolidation and to help you feel naturally sleepy at the right times.

Over time, as your sleep becomes more stable and refreshing, the time spent in bed is gradually increased to meet your body's needs. Though it may feel challenging at first, SRT can help reset your sleep patterns for long-term improvement.

How to do sleep restriction therapy (SRT):

Sleep restriction therapy is a targeted approach to improve sleep for those who struggle with insomnia. It might sound a bit backwards at first – sleep less to sleep better?

1. **Check if it's right for you:** First things first, make sure you have been diagnosed with insomnia. This therapy is specifically designed for those who have trouble falling or staying asleep.
2. **Establish a baseline:** Start by keeping a diary of your sleep for a week or two to see how much sleep you get each night. Let's say you average about six hours a night. That will be your starting target – but remember, never aim for less than 5.5 hours as that's not enough rest for most adults. I am aware that you might say 'I am getting less than that' but bear with this, the trick to this lies in the consolidation process and the forcing you to become sleepy. (If this idea feels anxiety-inducing, work on the anxiety before going anywhere near this practice.)
3. **Set a sleep schedule:** If you need to wake up at 7 a.m., plan to go to bed at 1 a.m. This may leave you with more waking hours, but the idea is to build up your sleepiness enough so that when it's finally time to hit the pillow, you fall asleep more easily and stay asleep.
4. **Gradually increase sleep time:** Once you start sleeping consistently during your allotted hours, you can slowly add more sleep time by 15–30 minutes each week, as long as you're still able to fall asleep within 20 minutes and stay asleep.

5. **Keep things consistent:** The key to making this work is consistency – especially when it comes to your wake-up time. Stick to the same time every morning, even at weekends. Get up, get lots of light and get moving to shake off sleepiness. This regularity helps your body clock sync up with your new sleep schedule.

Important

- **Understanding the process:** SRT helps to build up 'sleep pressure' (the natural urge to sleep) during the day, SRT helps you feel more tired and calm when it's finally time to sleep, making it easier to drift off.
- **Get back in sync:** SRT can help you get back in sync with your body's natural sleep–wake cycle. By limiting your time in bed, SRT trains your body to sleep at the right time, realigning your internal clock with when you go to bed. This helps you follow your body's natural signals for when it's time to feel sleepy and when it's time to wake up.
- **Safety first:** SRT is not suitable for everyone. It's especially important to avoid if your job requires alertness and precision, like driving or operating machinery, because the initial stages can make you extra sleepy during the day. It's important to speak with your GP or a sleep specialist to confirm if you have insomnia before trying this approach. They can offer guidance tailored to your specific sleep issues.

Thankfully, SRT isn't permanent – though many clients curse me while going through it! It's hard work, and yes, it can leave you feeling drained. But let's face it: you weren't feeling great to begin with. The difference now is that you're taking action, and the discomfort has a purpose. Many people see improvement within a week, though it can take longer. Once clients find their timing 'sweet spot', they often stick to it long-term because of how much better they feel. It's a tough process, but when it works the results are worth it.

Why do you fear sleep?

Why do sleep problems feel so overwhelming? Perhaps it's because sleep, a state where we relinquish control, occupies such a significant part of our lives. For those with hypervigilant minds, the tendency to ruminate or catastrophise can transform a restless night into a spiral of anxiety, where worst-case scenarios dominate and relaxation becomes impossible. Or maybe it's the vulnerability of surrendering to the unknown each night – or the profound loneliness of lying awake at 3 a.m., when sleep won't come.

Some clients have shared a few choice words with me when I suggest that broken or restless sleep can sometimes be expected – and I completely understand! There's a limit to what feels acceptable. On those mornings when you wake up feeling drained and far from refreshed, it's easy to blame sleep itself. But here's the truth: sleep is naturally variable. Stress, diet, physical activity and countless other factors can shape how restorative it feels. Not every night will leave you feeling recharged, and that's OK – it doesn't mean your sleep is broken. That said, if poor sleep becomes the rule rather than the exception, it's time to dig deeper and uncover what might be going on.

If you believe sleep must be perfect every night, any deviation from this ideal can create anxiety, reinforcing the idea that something is wrong. Ironically, this anxiety is often what makes sleep even harder to achieve.

Part of the problem can be in how sleep is portrayed in the media. Headlines about the supposed dangers of poor sleep often exaggerate findings, making people feel that even minor disturbances in sleep are disastrous. Take, for example, a study linking sleep problems to prostate cancer. It found that men who spent more than 30 minutes awake after going to bed had a 15–20 per cent higher risk of developing prostate cancer.[5] While this sounds alarming, the absolute risk remains low for most, and many factors beyond sleep, like genetics and lifestyle, contribute to cancer risk. Narrowing such findings into sleep-specific headlines can lead to unnecessary fear.

As someone who has worked in a sleep clinic, I've seen the impact of this firsthand. The day after a TV programme aired about the dangers of poor sleep, we'd often see a spike in anxious calls. Sensationalism can make something as natural as waking up during the night feel like a crisis.

Your brain, after all, is wired to protect you by alerting you to potential threats. It triggers stress and anxiety as part of your body's natural defence mechanism, preparing you to act quickly in the face of danger. However, in modern life, your brain can misinterpret non-life-threatening situations – like media headlines, work pressures, social conflicts or financial worries – as dangers, leaving you in a state of heightened vigilance. If your stress response is keeping you awake, it's doing exactly what it was designed to do: protect you. The key is to identify and address the triggers behind this stress so your brain can stand down from its protective guard.

Journalists have a tricky job balancing engagement with accuracy. But a little more care – like including study limitations or emphasising broader health contexts – could help prevent unnecessary anxiety. This would allow people to focus on what truly supports healthy sleep, rather than worrying over exaggerated risks.

The stages of sleep

Do you believe that once you fall asleep, you should stay asleep until morning without waking? In reality, it's completely natural to wake briefly during the night, particularly during transitions between sleep and especially between 3 and 4 a.m. Learning to accept and manage these awakenings can help you get back to sleep more easily rather than stressing about it.

If you use a sleep tracker, you've probably seen your sleep cycles represented as a hypnogram. This chart shows the different stages of sleep throughout the night, making it seem like each stage – wakefulness, non-REM (NREM) sleep and REM sleep – is distinct and separate. But in reality, the transitions between these stages are much more blurred.

On a typical night, most adults go through four to six sleep cycles, with each cycle consisting of various stages: N1 (stage 1: light sleep – the gateway to sleep), N2 (stage 2: light sleep), N3 (stage 3: deep sleep – the body's restoration phase). The average adult spends about 13–23 per cent of the night here and and approximately 20–25 per cent in REM sleep (rapid eye movement – the dreaming stage). These sleep cycles repeat every 90 to 120 minutes. Early in the night, your body prioritises NREM sleep, especially the deeply restorative N3 stage. As the night progresses, REM sleep takes over, playing a larger role in each subsequent cycle.

Your sleep pattern, or 'sleep architecture', naturally shifts as you age. While you can't control exactly when you enter deep sleep or REM, spending enough time in bed increases the chances that your body will cycle through these critical stages.

This is where sleep duration recommendations – typically seven to nine hours for most adults – help. These guidelines aren't just about getting enough sleep but ensuring you have enough time in bed for your body to naturally progress through all the stages of sleep. Even though you can't directly control when these stages occur, following the recommendations improves the likelihood that your body will get the deep, restorative rest it needs (see Appendix for more details).

Always remember that these recommendations are merely a starting point, as sleep needs can vary greatly from person to person. The most reliable measure of your sleep quality is not a number but how rested, refreshed and energised you feel during the day.[6]

N1 (stage 1 NREM sleep)

N1, or stage 1 of NREM sleep, typically makes up about 1–5 per cent of an adult's total sleep, and it represents the transition from wakefulness to sleep. It's the lightest stage, typically lasting for just a few minutes (1–7 minutes on average), and can be easily disrupted, causing you to wake up.

During this stage, there is a decrease in muscle tone throughout the body, though muscles are not fully relaxed. Brain activity begins to slow, from wakeful alpha to lower-frequency theta waves, indicating a relaxed state. You start to lose awareness of your surroundings, making this stage a buffer against the sensory input of the external world.

N2 (stage 2 NREM sleep)

N2, or stage 2 of NREM sleep, typically makes up about 45–50 per cent of an adult's total sleep. During N2 sleep, the brain produces a series of specific patterns: sleep spindles, which are sudden bursts of oscillatory brain activity, and K-complexes, which are single, large waves. These patterns are thought to play roles in consolidating memories and protecting sleep from external disturbances.

Both heart rate and body temperature drop, further relaxing the body and preparing it for the deeper sleep stages. Muscle tone throughout the body reduces further, though it is not as low as in the deepest sleep stage. N2 sleep is a vital stage of the sleep cycle that contributes significantly to physical and mental restoration, cognitive function, memory consolidation and overall health.

Am I awake, or am I asleep?

Light sleep often doesn't get as much attention as deep sleep or REM, but it's vital to your nightly rest. It serves as the bridge that helps you transition from wakefulness into the deeper, more restorative stage of sleep. However, N2 can be deceptive. During N2, your brain activity slows and your body begins to relax, but it's not uncommon to feel a heightened sense of alertness. You can feel you're still awake, even when you've already crossed the 'sleep barrier'.

This is the territory of paradoxical insomnia, also called sleep state misperception, where you feel like you're barely sleeping, even though sleep studies show you're getting a relatively normal amount of rest. It's a peculiar phenomenon because, in these cases, the actual sleep architecture of someone with paradoxical insomnia is often very similar to that of a good sleeper.[7] Research suggests that it may affect about 5–10 per cent of people with insomnia, though exact prevalence rates vary depending on the population and diagnostic criteria. It's generally more common in individuals who experience chronic insomnia, anxiety or heightened emotional arousal.

Learning about sleep state misperception can be a relief. If you've spent years feeling like you don't sleep, finding that your body is getting more rest than you thought can be comforting. Also, knowing that lighter stages of sleep, like N1 and N2, still contribute to your overall recovery can reduce the anxiety that comes from the experience. This shift in perspective often helps people stop fighting sleep and instead embrace a more relaxed, accepting approach towards their sleep experience.

However, there is a problematic flip side: learning about sleep state misperception can also be deeply upsetting. If you feel chronically exhausted, finding out you are technically sleeping but still feel terrible can feel invalidating or even dismissive of your experience.

Meet Alfie. Following a sleep study, after years of being convinced he barely slept, the results told a different tale. 'But I felt awake most of the time!' Alfie exclaimed, puzzled.

For Alfie, it was a lightbulb moment when he discovered he was sleeping more than he thought. Understanding that it's normal to feel awake during lighter sleep stages can be comforting. However, this doesn't mean Alfie's struggles with sleep aren't real. Sleep state misperception can be tied to deeper issues like anxiety, depression or stress.

The next time you think you haven't slept, remind yourself that N2, this 'in-between' stage, can feel quite wakeful as it leads you into the deeper, more restorative stages of sleep. You are getting rest, even if it doesn't feel like the deep slumber you might expect.

It's completely understandable to feel frustrated or upset if this is happening to you. Even though your body may be getting more rest than you think, the fact that you still feel exhausted is real and deserves attention to ensure nothing else is going on.

It's about understanding that sleep isn't the whole picture. Other factors, like stress, anxiety or even physical conditions, could be influencing how you feel, and you can work on these. Why are you a light sleeper?

The answer to why some people have lighter sleep and don't feel as rested involves a mix of genes, the body's ability to handle stress, a person's daily habits and even the history of human survival. It might also have something to do with the weird phenomenon of local sleep, where certain parts of the brain exhibit sleep-like activity patterns while the rest remain awake. It's a fascinating aspect of brain function that highlights the complexity of sleep regulation and suggests different brain regions can have varying levels of arousal or restfulness at any given time.

- Some people might naturally have lighter sleep or wake up more quickly because of their genetic makeup.
- When stressed, the body goes into alert mode, producing stress hormones that can make it hard to fall into deep, restful sleep.
- What you do during the day significantly affects your night; how much you exercise, what you eat and exposure to light can affect sleep.
- From an evolutionary standpoint, light sleep might have been helpful for early humans to stay alert to dangers in their environment, allowing them to wake up quickly if needed. This trait might still affect some people's sleep patterns today – think of new parents who often sleep more lightly because their brain is 'listening'.
- Specific health issues can also disrupt our sleep, causing more light sleep or making us wake up more often.

N3 (stage 3 NREM sleep), also known as slow-wave sleep (SWS)

After about 20 minutes, heart rate and body temperature drop as you fall into N3 sleep, also known as deep or slow-wave sleep (SWS). It's like the brain's quiet time and is believed to be the most restful form of sleep, typically making up about 20 per cent of an adult's total sleep.[8] Brain waves slow down, creating significant, slow patterns called delta waves. N3 is when the body goes into repair and sort mode, producing growth hormone for bodily repair and sifting through memories, filing and cataloguing the story of your day. This deep sleep usually lasts 20–30 minutes, especially in the first part of the night. You then move back up through N2 and up into REM sleep. After a bad night's sleep, your brain works hard to catch up on the deep sleep you missed. That's why you often sleep much better and more deeply the next night.

A commonly held but misleading belief is that 'an hour of sleep before midnight is worth two after'. The truth is that the most restorative sleep occurs during the first third of your sleep period, no matter when you go to bed. No matter if you settle down to sleep at 9 p.m. or

2 a.m., you will usually experience most of your deep, restorative rest during the early part of your sleep period.[9] Due to individual chronotypes, not everyone is inclined to sleep early. If you're a night owl, you're unlikely to be in bed before midnight. What's important is aligning your sleep schedule with your own circadian rhythm to ensure you're receiving restorative sleep during the initial phases of your sleep cycle. Children and teens get the most deep sleep because they are growing rapidly. Many adults often wish they could sleep like they did in their youth, but sorry – sleep naturally changes with age.

REM sleep

During REM, the body rests, but the mind is intensely active, engaged in critical tasks: consolidating memories, processing emotions and fostering creativity. In fact, during this stage, the brain is nearly as active as when we're awake, a physiological paradox that hints at how vital it is to our overall wellbeing.

REM sleep is characterised by rapid eye movements, muscle relaxation, irregular breathing and an elevated heart rate. Brain activity during this stage mirrors wakefulness. Newborns typically spend about eight hours in REM, making up half of their total sleep. For adults, REM occupies roughly 25 per cent of total sleep time. For someone sleeping seven to eight hours, this amounts to around 90–120 minutes of REM. Falling slightly below two hours of REM is still within the normal range for most adults, with natural fluctuations occurring each night.

The quality of sleep, and whether it's considered 'good' or 'bad', largely depend on how you feel during the day and the overall quality of your sleep. A frequent issue for many is waking up between 3–4 a.m. and struggling to fall back asleep. It's important to understand that it can be quite normal but can happen for a multitude of reasons. These can range from stress and anxiety to changes in your schedule – like having to wake up earlier – which can unintentionally disrupt your sleep patterns. Other factors might include hormonal fluctuations, environmental disturbances, dietary choices or even the natural progression of your sleep cycles. There are many reasons why this might occur, and we'll explore them in detail later on. Abruptly cutting REM sleep – due to an alarm going off, for example – can take a serious toll on your brain, affecting key functions like memory consolidation, emotional regulation, and creativity.[10] If you miss out on it, you're likely to feel emotionally off, less empathetic and more reactive the next day.

Everyone has dreams, but not everyone remembers them – 80 per cent of people who wake up during REM sleep will briefly recall their dreams before the content floats away.

Having vivid dreams, especially after a stressful day, might be your brain's way of finding balance. A 2009 study showed that REM sleep helps manage stress. The dreams you remember from REM sleep are part of the brain's way of coping with stress. Sometimes, these dreams can be disturbing when you're *really* stressed.[11] REM sleep acts like a mental rehearsal space where your brain practises dealing with complex emotions and situations, preparing you for real life.

When stressed, your body doesn't simply 'turn off' at night. It remains hypervigilant, in a state of heightened alertness that doesn't just disappear when your head hits the pillow. This alertness can bleed into the sleep cycle, particularly into REM. Instead of using this critical stage for emotional processing and memory consolidation, your brain – still on high alert – continues scanning for danger, even though there's no immediate threat.

The result? Nightmares. Disturbing dreams. It's as if your brain, unable to let go of the day's stress, amplifies emotional experiences during sleep. These heightened emotional responses aren't random; they reflect the mind's desperate attempt to make sense of unresolved tension and anxiety. The more stress you experience, the more intense and fragmented your dreams become. And, as many clients tell me, it's not uncommon to wake up feeling just as exhausted as when they went to bed. This is the insidious cycle of stress and sleep: stress disrupts sleep, poor sleep increases stress, and round and round it goes.

Nightmares and night terrors

There is emerging evidence suggesting that nightmares and disturbed dreaming might be associated with certain health conditions, including autoimmune diseases like lupus (SLE). A recent study explored the relationship between sleep, inflammation and cognitive disturbances in lupus patients.[12] Participants reported symptoms such as fatigue, mental fog and emotional challenges, which often coincided with or preceded disease flares. Notably, 43 per cent of patients experienced vivid, sometimes unsettling dreams that disrupted their sleep.

While these findings raise the possibility that nightmares could serve as an early warning sign of an impending lupus flare, this connection is far from conclusive. The study hypothesised that inflammation in the brain might affect REM sleep, reducing its ability to process emotions and amplifying perceived threats during dreaming. For some, this could manifest as unsettling scenarios in their dreams.

If this link is confirmed through further research, it might provide a valuable tool for early intervention, helping patients and healthcare providers anticipate and manage flares. However, it's important to remember that nightmares are common and often unrelated to any medical condition.

So, while it's interesting, it needs more research before it can be taken as definitive. The last thing I want is to overemphasise this potential association and inadvertently increase anxiety around sleep. In my work with clients struggling with insomnia, I frequently encounter health anxiety – a tendency to become hyper-focused on bodily symptoms, which can make matters worse. The amygdala, the part of the brain that deals with emotion, is always listening. If we direct too much attention towards potential health issues, it will latch on to that fear, keeping the body in a heightened state of alertness, making restful sleep even more elusive.

Put simply, while nightmares might one day help us spot early signs of autoimmune flares, we need to be cautious. Mistaking normal sleep disturbances for signs of illness could increase anxiety and worsen insomnia, especially for those already feeling stressed. Can you take a balanced approach – keeping an eye on patterns without letting worry become another reason for sleepless nights?

When a nightmare is a sign of emotional overload

While nightmares might sometimes act as an early warning sign in other cases, they may result from strong emotional reactions. Sacha has been wrestling with nightmares for a while now. Though the details often escape her, one particularly persistent scenario refuses to fade away. In our session, she shares a recurring nightmare involving a stalker. 'I wake up in a panic and then I can't get back to sleep because I'm too scared.

I can't get out of bed as I feel the presence of this person. I just lie there for hours, sweating it out until it's time to get up.' This terrifying dream has been haunting her for months, severely disrupting her sleep.

When you experience something distressing, your mind often dreams about it as a natural mechanism for processing and resolving traumatic memories. Research shows that REM sleep when most vivid dreaming occurs is required for the consolidation of procedural and emotional memories.[13] Added to that, during REM sleep, levels of the stress-related chemical norepinephrine (noradrenaline) are reduced, which allows for the safe re-processing of emotional memories.[14]

Nightmares and other sleep disturbances are dreams that have become 'stuck', often repeating because the brain's creative resources are exhausted. This phenomenon is partly due to the amygdala, which becomes highly active in response to emotionally charged content. Consequently, the brain continually revisits these distressing scenarios in an attempt to process and resolve the underlying emotions. Without effective resolution, however, the cycle persists. The brain's efforts, though well intentioned, can sometimes feel counterproductive. Isn't it remarkable how the brain tries to help, even if it doesn't always succeed in the most helpful way?

There are various ways to work to resolve nightmares, Dr Justin Havens has developed a powerful tool – Dream Completion Technique® (DCT) – that can stop nightmares in their tracks.[15] It is an active transformation that helps rewire the brain's response to traumatic memories without reliving the trauma, which can be distressing.

You have more influence over your dreams than you might realise, as we will see later regarding lucid dreaming. Dreams originate in the subconscious mind, which operates differently from the conscious mind. Changing beliefs at this level requires more than conscious effort; it often needs therapeutic interventions of techniques like DCT. Finding a way to truly believe that 'there is nothing to fear in your dream' – that whatever happened, no matter how awful, is now just a dream – is key to releasing the hold it might have over you, even though it's challenging.

What's fascinating about Sacha's dream is that it is a complete construct, and she has no idea where this stalker nightmare originated. Thankfully, she has never encountered a real stalker.

I ask Sacha if we can focus on the most recent nightmare – not relive the entire experience (which is essential, as I don't want to re-traumatise her); can she just think about the moment she woke up and what she would like to happen next that feels good, something that would make her feel safe and empowered? Anything can happen in your dream – it is yours to create a scenario where you are whatever or whoever you need to be.

Sacha appears doubtful but ventures, 'I'd wear massive steel boots that I can grind people into the ground with and then I would become huge, bigger than the buildings, as I stride off down the street like a powerful warrior princess walking away, having won the battle.'

We get into her idea, having some fun with it, making it bigger and more intense, diving deeper than the dream was at the point of waking. Something interesting happens – I can see her doubts begin to dissipate as she allows herself to fully embrace her vision. There is an almost imperceptible straightening of her spine, a tilt of her head as her eyes widen – she's in control; she's got this. Sacha's voice, now steady and commanding, declares, 'I will wear those boots,' her tone leaving no room for doubt. 'And with each step, I will tell him he cannot stalk me anymore.' It's a curious moment, as I can see that Sacha is not merely envisioning a scene; she is meeting something unknown from her unconscious mind.

It demonstrates how quickly the mind can create vivid, empowering scenarios just as it generates nightmares. This act of transformation is potent. By envisioning herself as a warrior princess who can defeat her stalker, Sacha rewires her subconscious to feel safer and more in control.

I encourage Sacha to continue developing her idea. Before she goes to sleep that night, she should revisit this scenario and prime her dream process by stocking her 'dream shelf' with things that will enable the dream to be completed.

The Dream Completion Technique® empowers you by giving you control over your dreams.[16] It alleviates the fear and anxiety that nightmares can cause, fostering emotional regulation and promoting a peaceful sleep. If your dream idea doesn't work, come up with another idea for your 'dream shelf', remembering that its emotional intensity must match or exceed that of the dream at the point of waking. Turn this practice into a habit – you are teaching your brain to sleep through anything, which is its natural state. Don't give up until you are sleeping peacefully through the night.

Night terrors

Night terrors differ from nightmares in several key ways. First, it is more likely to be your bed partner or family who experience you having one. During a night terror, you might suddenly sit upright in bed, scream, thrash about and appear highly distressed. You may also sweat, experience a rapid heartbeat and be hard to comfort or awaken. Unlike nightmares – which happen during REM sleep and are often remembered – those who experience night terrors typically have no recollection of the episode the next day.

Night terrors are most common in children aged three to seven, although they can affect adults as well. Triggers include stress, lack of sleep, fever or certain medications, though the exact cause is not always understood.

If your bed partner or child is waking due to night terrors, stay calm and resist the urge to wake them; instead, focus on ensuring their safety. Gently guide them away from anything that could cause harm, but don't restrain them. Soft words, a gentle touch – these can sometimes ease the intensity of the episode, though the person may not respond or even remember the event come morning.

After the storm passes, allow them to return to sleep naturally. There's no need for deep discussions the next day – night terrors are rarely remembered, and revisiting the details might only create unnecessary anxiety.

Tips to prevent night terrors

- Keep regular bedtimes and ensure enough sleep.
- Use relaxation techniques like deep breathing before bed.

- Limit caffeine, sugar and screen time before sleep.
- Address triggers: treat medical issues, manage stress and avoid sleep deprivation.
- Try scheduled awakenings: wake the person briefly before typical episodes.
- Consult a sleep specialist for persistent issues.

Summary

This chapter invited you to take a fresh look at your relationship with sleep. It's not just about avoiding caffeine or putting your phone away before bed; good sleep goes far beyond the basics.

How you spend your day plays a powerful role in how easily you drift into sleep at night. By focusing on these daytime rhythms, you can take some of the pressure off the act of sleeping itself. Sleep is a friend, not an enemy. Approaching it with curiosity and kindness, rather than fear and frustration, can transform your experience. Even the imperfections – nights of wakefulness or moments of restlessness – are part of sleep's natural ebb and flow.

We looked at the forces that shape your rest: your body's internal clock, the balance of sleep pressure (the gradual build-up of your need for rest over the day, known as Process S) and circadian timing (your body's natural daily rhythms, or Process C), and how these processes prove that biologically you can sleep.

But when sleep goes 'off' – you're battling anxiety, lying awake for hours or waking from vivid nightmares – it's easy to feel like something's wrong with you. These moments aren't signs of failure. More often than not, they're logical responses to stress, misaligned schedules or external pressures – not personal flaws.

This is an invitation to step back from the frustration and fear surrounding sleep. Instead, see it for what it is: a deeply human, sometimes messy, but ultimately supportive part of your life. What if you treated sleep like a best friend – can you accept it, even when it's not perfect?

Actionable steps

- It's normal to wake up once or twice during the night. You may need to pee, then lie there for a bit, and then calmly drop off. If this isn't happening, get up and do something you enjoy – try not to get wound up.
- Reduce stressors by practising relaxation techniques such as mindfulness or deep breathing throughout the day.
- Reframe your relationship with sleep by viewing it as a natural and supportive process.
- Remember, nightmares or restless nights aren't purely random. They often reflect the mind's attempt to process unresolved emotions, yet factors like illness and medication, and wider mental health challenges like PTSD, can also contribute.
- Techniques like sleep restriction therapy (SRT) or Dream Completion Technique® give you practical ways to work with your body, not against it.
- Accept that waking briefly during the night is normal; avoid clock-watching if you can't fall back asleep.

CHAPTER TWO

A gradual, natural process

It's possible to enjoy, even love falling asleep

When drifting off at night feels like stepping into the danger zone – laden with tension, anticipation and the lingering echoes of the day – you might find yourself longing for a swift, all-encompassing escape from the thoughts that crowd your mind. Yet, much like any intimate experience, there is another way to approach this nightly ritual.

How quickly you fall asleep, or as Dr Chris Winter calls it, your 'speed to unconsciousness',[1] is influenced by a constellation of factors. Sleepiness/sleep pressure gets obstructed by worry, anxiety and stress. And on top of that, external influences like life, sugar, caffeine, alcohol, your environment, health conditions and sleep timing play significant roles in either inviting sleep in or chasing it away. Shift workers who have a tendency towards sleep deprivation often fall asleep incredibly quickly.

When you're reading this, your brain is likely producing higher-frequency beta waves (wave frequency decreases from gamma to beta, then alpha, theta and finally delta), which are associated with focused thinking and problem-solving. As you start to relax – maybe pausing between chapters or just daydreaming a little – your brain begins to shift gears, producing alpha waves that are connected to calm, lightly meditative states. This transition helps your brain to synchronise better, promoting relaxation and preparing you for sleep if you're heading to bed.

If you relax even further – maybe you put the book down and let your thoughts wander – you might start to experience theta waves, which signal deep relaxation, the kind you feel right before falling asleep. Theta waves are linked with the subconscious mind, where unexpected connections and insights can surface, and creativity and intuition often come alive. This is the process of falling asleep and happens in reverse when we wake up naturally.

The hypnagogic state is a bit like the flow state, where you're completely absorbed in an activity, but with a key difference: flow involves active engagement and a sense of control, while the hypnagogic state is more about letting your mind wander freely. This twilight of consciousness is fleeting, and many of us miss its magic altogether. Some even find it a little unsettling. But for those who tune in as they drift off, it offers a captivating glimpse into an inner world. The hypnopompic state is essentially the reverse of the hypnagogic state, happening in the moments of waking up. It can involve vivid imagery, fragmented thoughts or even lingering sensations from dreams.

Interestingly, research shows that the hypnagogic state may play a role in problem-solving and memory consolidation. It's like your brain is decluttering, making space for new connections and insights.[2]

A lot is happening with your brain's neurotransmitters as you move from wakefulness into the hypnagogic state – the dreamy in-between phase. Levels of acetylcholine, a neurotransmitter that enhances vivid mental imagery, begin to rise, helping create the striking, dream-like visuals often experienced in this state. At the same time, serotonin, which helps regulate mood, and norepinephrine, which supports alertness and arousal, both decrease, allowing your mind to relax and let go of wakeful tension. Meanwhile, GABA (gamma-aminobutyric acid), the brain's calming neurotransmitter, increases. This helps quieten down overactive brain activity and smooths the transition into deeper relaxation.

These changes in your brain chemistry work together to create a state that feels calm yet creatively rich, where vivid thoughts and images begin to flow effortlessly.

While this state doesn't provide the deep, restorative rest of slow-wave sleep, it offers a form of mental rest and relaxation that's valuable and ripe with creativity. Spending a little time in the hypnagogic state can ease tension, spark creativity and prepare your mind for deeper sleep. It's something you might even start looking forward to.

What I'm really describing is the same process as falling asleep. In sleep, this would lead to deep rest. But if you're reading, you might just put the book down and carry on with your day, hopefully feeling a bit more relaxed. Finding this state of calm – whether you're reading, listening to a yoga nidra or gazing out the window on a long train journey – allows your mind to drift freely and release tension. It's a space where you can simply exist without effort – a rare kind of freedom in our busy lives.

In the morning, the hypnagogic state has a twin, known as the hypnopompic state, which you experience in those fleeting moments of waking. It's when the veil between dreams and reality is thin, letting the dream world slide into the edges of waking life. As you wake, you might find yourself grasping at the fading echoes of a dream, caught in that delicate limbo between two realms.

These states aren't just curiosities – they're sought by meditators, whose practice allows them to enter theta states while maintaining awareness of being in a meditative state, allowing them to observe their thoughts and sensations without getting completely absorbed by them.

It's also the realm of lucid dreamers, who explore and even control their dream environments. By embracing the fluidity of these moments, they embark on conscious dream adventures that blend the edges between sleep and wakefulness.

Ultimately, understanding and embracing these transitional states can transform how you feel about sleep. Instead of dreading the process, you might find yourself looking forward to it, discovering that falling asleep can become one of life's greatest pleasures.

Tip

Keeping a notebook by your bed can be helpful to jot down any interesting thoughts that arise in these states. And don't worry – writing them down won't wake you up. In fact, it can help reassure your brain that you've 'parked' the thought, making it easier to fall back asleep afterwards.

Lucid dreaming

Lucid dreaming is where you become aware that you are dreaming while still within the dream. You might find yourself thinking, 'I'm dreaming!' or 'This is a dream!' This realisation often, but not always, allows you to control your actions and navigate the dream environment intentionally and consciously.

Charlie Morley, a lucid dreaming expert, often speaks about the transformative potential of these states. In his teachings, Morley emphasises how the hypnagogic state is a gateway to lucid dreaming, offering a unique space for creativity, problem-solving and personal growth.

His work extends beyond the fascination with dream control and dives into the therapeutic benefits of lucid dreaming. The journal *Traumatology* published the results of a ground-breaking peer-reviewed scientific study on lucid dreaming to reduce PTSD symptoms as developed by Morley.[3] He explains that you can confront and transform traumatic memories in a safe and controlled environment by becoming aware within your dreams.

The results of the study were highly significant, with the average PTSD score dropping below the PTSD threshold by the end of the week-long study.

Morley highlights that the hypnagogic state, where the mind is particularly receptive to suggestion and visualisation, is an effective time to practise lucid dreaming induction techniques. These techniques often involve setting intentions, performing reality checks, and using affirmations to enhance dream awareness.

In the past, lucid dreaming was thought to be purely a product of imagination. However, recent studies provide evidence of its neurological basis. In one small study, participants who were experienced lucid dreamers underwent functional MRI scans.[4] They were able to signal when they were lucid dreaming by making specific eye movements and clenching their hands within the dream. The corresponding brain areas responsible for hand movement lit up, demonstrating that lucid dreaming involves real neural activity.

While the study has its limitations, its innovative approach opens new avenues for exploring the complex interplay between sleep, consciousness, and brain activity. This research offers a deeper understanding of the neural processes involved in lucid dreaming, confirming that it's more than just vivid imagination.

Hallucinations, jerks, paralysis and exploding head syndrome

There is a truth that not everything about the moments just before you fall asleep or just after you wake up is pleasant. During these transitional times – the hypnagogic state (falling asleep) and the hypnopompic state (waking up) – you might experience phenomena such as vivid dreams, known as hypnagogic or hypnopompic hallucinations, and frightening and surprisingly common events like sleep paralysis.

Hypnagogic and hypnopompic hallucinations are vivid sensory experiences or jerks (hypnic jerks) that happen as you drift off to sleep or wake up. These can include seeing shapes, hearing sounds or feeling sensations that aren't really there. While these hallucinations can be unnerving, they are generally harmless and often linked to irregular sleep patterns or conditions like narcolepsy.

Sleep paralysis happens when you find yourself unable to move or speak, even though you can still breathe. It is a very common occurrence, especially in people with narcolepsy, a sleep disorder that causes excessive daytime sleepiness and sudden loss of muscle tone. It can happen as you fall asleep or wake up. While they can be scary, hypnagogic and hypnopompic hallucinations and sleep paralysis are typically harmless – it can be the fear of them that makes them worse.

Historically, sleep paralysis has been widely misunderstood and often attributed to supernatural forces. In Western folklore, the entity responsible was frequently referred to as an 'incubus' or a 'nightmare.' Interestingly, the term *nightmare* was originally described not as a bad dream but as a demonic figure believed to sit on the sleeper's chest, causing feelings of suffocation and intense fear. The incubus was said to torment men, while a succubus targeted women, with both entities thought to attack during the night.

Different cultures have other interpretations of this unsettling phenomenon. In Japanese folklore, the paralysis is blamed on a vengeful spirit called *kanashibari*, meaning 'bound in metal', which leaves the victim immobilised. Even literature reflects this fear: in Bram Stoker's *Dracula*, Lucy experiences a similar sensation – a crushing weight on her chest, rendering her unable to scream or move, capturing the eerie helplessness of sleep paralysis.

Another startling and very unnerving phenomenon is exploding head syndrome (EHS),[5] where you might hear a loud, startling noise as you're falling asleep or waking up. Though the sound can be shocking, it's entirely imagined – created by your brain. EHS is less common than other hypnagogic experiences, such as brief visual or auditory sensations that occur as you drift off. You could think of EHS as a more intense version of these auditory states, where your mind conjures a sudden, loud noise just as you transition into or out of sleep.

All of these states can be intensified by stress or stimulant intake, including caffeine and nicotine. Fearing that these sensations are something more sinister can heighten anxiety and make the experiences even more unsettling. In her book *Night Terrors: Troubled Sleep and the Stories We Tell About It*, Alice Vernon details her own encounters with the hypnagogic state, describing it as a 'twilight zone' where the boundaries between reality and dreams blur disturbingly.[6] She recounts vivid and often frightening hypnagogic hallucinations – images and sounds that seem real but are conjured by the mind during this transitional phase.

Vernon explains that these hallucinations can be deeply unsettling, sometimes making you question your sanity. This reaction occurs because our minds are wired to perceive threats in ambiguous situations – a survival mechanism. For example, a simple muscle twitch might feel like falling from a height, or a shadow might appear as a threatening figure.

Recognising that these things are natural, though sometimes startling, parts of the sleep process can be reassuring. Remember that experiencing these phenomena doesn't mean you're losing your mind; they are simply your brain's way of navigating the transition between sleep and wakefulness and are a natural part of the sleep process. By managing stress, avoiding stimulants and remembering that these sensations are harmless, you can minimise their impact, and while I really do appreciate that these can be frightening things to experience, you can maintain peace of mind.

> ## Unexpected movement
>
> While hypnic jerks, restless leg syndrome (RLS) and periodic limb movement disorder (PLMD) all involve sleep-related movements (see page 248), they differ in timing, causes, sensations and their impact on sleep quality. Hypnic jerks are brief and happen as you fall asleep. RLS involves uncomfortable sensations and an irresistible urge to move the legs while awake, and PLMD consists of involuntary leg (and even body) movements during sleep.

Waking up tired: sleep inertia

Have you ever woken up and felt as though your body was pulling you back into the depths of sleep? That groggy, sluggish state is what we call sleep inertia. It's not about laziness or a lack of motivation. It's your brain, caught between two worlds: sleep and wakefulness.

This phenomenon is universal, yet deeply personal. For some, it's fleeting, gone in 15 minutes. For others, it lingers for up to two hours,[7] a fog that refuses to lift. Why does this happen? It's not just about how much sleep you get, but when you wake up. If your alarm jars you out of deep sleep, you're bound to feel disoriented, no matter how many hours you've logged. Sleep inertia is the result of your brain transitioning from deep sleep to full wakefulness – a natural biological process meant to protect your rest and conserve energy.

For night owls, this struggle is even more pronounced. Their bodies are wired to sleep and wake later, so when the world demands an early start, they're forced to wake during their biological night – the time their brains are least prepared to function. The result? Sleep inertia feels heavier, harder to shake.

And for teens, it's an almost inevitable battle. During adolescence, the body's natural sleep–wake rhythm shifts later, meaning teens are biologically programmed to fall asleep and wake up later than adults. But school schedules don't accommodate this shift. Instead, they demand early mornings that cut short sleep cycles and force teens into their days before their brains are ready. The result? Chronic grogginess, impaired focus and a tougher time regulating emotions – all at a time when their developing minds need clarity and calm the most.

And then there's the snooze button, tempting you with promises of just a little more rest. But those extra minutes can backfire, plunging you into another cycle of deep sleep, only to be interrupted again. It's a reminder that sometimes, what we think will soothe us can make things worse.

For teens, night owls, shift workers, and anyone navigating irregular schedules, this grogginess can feel like a daily battle. But there's hope. A splash of cold water to the face[8] and rehydrating with a glass of water can help the brain and body shift gears. Activities like exposure to bright light and light movement signal to your brain to release wake-promoting hormones like cortisol, helping you feel more alert. Over time, aligning your sleep with your natural rhythms can make a meaningful difference.

Waking at the same time every day trains your internal clock to expect wakefulness at that hour, reducing grogginess over time. Using a sunrise clock – which gradually brightens to simulate sunrise – instead of a loud alarm can help you wake more gently. While these strategies can help most people, individual responses may vary. If you frequently struggle with extreme grogginess or excessive fatigue despite trying these techniques, it may be worth consulting a sleep specialist to rule out conditions like sleep apnea or chronic sleep deprivation.

Sleep inertia isn't something to fight or fear. It's a sign that your body is doing its job – protecting your rest, preserving your energy. The key is to work with it, not against it, to create a gentler transition from rest to wakefulness. For teens especially, the challenge isn't just about sleep – it's about the social systems that need adjustment to accommodate this biological issue.

How much sleep do you need?

Ideally, you'd sleep until you felt refreshed, timing it to suit your needs. However, sleep beliefs, shaped by personal experiences and societal norms, often lead to chasing the elusive 'perfect' sleep. The notion of needing eight hours of sleep stems from the Industrial Revolution's eight-hour work shift structure. While research suggests adults require seven to nine hours of sleep, individual needs vary. Quality trumps quantity; getting six or seven hours of restful sleep is better than tossing and turning for eight hours. Some thrive on less, while others need more.

Sociological research into tribes and communities that remain active after dark reveals fascinating insights into sleep duration. Dr Jerry Siegel, a professor of psychiatry at UCLA, and his team studied sleep in three pre-industrial societies – groups that live without modern technology like electricity – and found that people in these groups slept in one block (monophasic) for about 5.7 to 7.1 hours each night and got around an hour more between summer and winter.[9] Interestingly, these groups don't even have a word for insomnia in their languages, so the researchers had to explain what it means. In these groups, about 5 per cent occasionally had trouble falling asleep, and 9 per cent sometimes woke up during the night. However, only 1.5 per cent had frequent issues falling asleep, and 2.5 per cent regularly struggled with staying asleep. These rates are much lower than the 10 per cent to 30 per cent of people in industrialised societies who suffer from chronic insomnia.

Assuming everyone needs the same amount of sleep is a problem, as is comparing the way you sleep with the way others sleep. Insights from a comprehensive study involving over a million participants over six years help prove this point, revealing lower mortality rates among those who sleep six to seven hours.[10]

Too much or too little

Research shows that both too little sleep (less than six hours) and too much sleep (more than nine hours) are often linked to long-term health problems. It's important to recognise and prioritise the sleep needs and timing that work best for you.

The eight-hour myth
Rather than rigidly adhering to the eight-hour rule, focus on listening to your body, maintaining consistent sleep timing and allowing yourself

the time you need to sleep. Meet Jaivik; he is 35, lives alone and works two days a week in the office and three days at home in a support role for the military. He has had issues with his sleep for a while and has told me about many strategies he's tried without success. His GP has diagnosed insomnia, but Jaivik struggled with this and has seen many different specialists as he believed that there was something 'wrong' with him. But despite extensive testing, nothing has been found, and the insomnia diagnosis remains. Sitting across from me, he shared, 'I need a solid eight hours of sleep to function. Now I'm barely hitting six, and it's getting to me.'

He continued, 'It's like being in a constant mental fog and my brain isn't working. My thoughts aren't as sharp, and I struggle with stuff that used to come easily.' His stress levels were high; his internal narrative had become one of continual self-reproach; each night of insufficient rest felt like a personal shortfall, adding to a cycle of anxiety that only exacerbated his sleep challenges.

I was curious about his belief. 'Why do you think you need eight hours?' I asked. Jaivik seemed unsure: 'Isn't that what I need to optimise my performance?' It felt like a key turning in a lock – what does 'optimising my performance' mean to him?

The trend of optimising performance – whether through rigid schedules or self-quantification – often does more harm than good, setting you up to fail. In our relentless pursuit of optimisation, we tend to forget a fundamental truth: as I said previously, you are not a machine. Your energy and focus naturally ebb and flow, and what works for one person might not work for you. The stress that comes from constantly trying to meet some external metric can be counterproductive, increasing anxiety and disrupting your natural rhythms.

The pressure to perform at a high level all the time doesn't just undermine your wellbeing – it often ends up diminishing your overall productivity. The myth of perfect performance suggests there's a flawless formula for success, a one-size-fits-all approach that promises to unlock your full potential. But I call BS on that. Your biological rhythms are complex and unique to you, and their natural rise and fall are essential to your health. What optimises one person's life might not work for another, because optimisation is personal. True wellbeing comes from understanding and honouring your own rhythms, not forcing yourself into someone else's idea of perfection.

Jaivik's story is a testament to the weight external beliefs can place on us and the problem with a rigid goal based on an impossible target. Focusing solely on strict protocols or idealised numbers without considering the broader context of your life – work stress, environmental conditions, social relationships and lifestyle choices – can lead to a narrow approach that misses the root causes of sleep issues. With Jaivik, we decided to work on the bigger picture by keeping a sleep diary with the primary focus shifting from not how well he slept last night to the broader picture of his sleep quality over the past week or month.[11] There was other work we needed to do – his approach revealed insomnia's best friends, perfectionism and a high need to control life. Both were helpful traits in his work life, but not when it came to his sleep.

Sleep diaries

Keeping a sleep diary can help you understand your sleep patterns and needs. There are pros and cons to doing this: sleep diaries can become problematic if you get too focused on them. On the other hand, they can be helpful as they give you hard evidence to challenge your beliefs about how you have been sleeping. We often can believe the worst about sleep – we focus on the negative, not realising that it might not be as bad as we tell ourselves. Keeping a diary means you can't argue with your own evidence.

How to keep a sleep diary:

- **Paper diary:** You can keep a traditional paper sleep diary. Simply jot down key details each morning and evening, such as when you went to bed, how long it took to fall asleep, how many times you woke up during the night and how you felt upon waking.
- **Online or app-based diaries:** If you prefer a digital approach, there are many online tools and apps available.

Look for a 'consensus sleep diary' for the most accurate tracking. These are standardised and designed by sleep experts to give you and your healthcare provider a clear picture of your sleep patterns.

- **Apps:** There are apps like 'Sleepio', 'Sleepstation' and 'SleepScore' that offer sleep tracking features. Look for one that includes a daily journal feature where you can input your sleep details.
- **Medical websites:** Reputable sites like the NHS, Mayo Clinic or sleep research centres often provide downloadable or online sleep diaries that you can use.
- **Consistency is key:** Record your sleep patterns daily for at least one to two weeks, stay consistent and be honest with your answers. This will provide enough data to identify trends or issues.

Once you've kept your diary for a few weeks, share it with your GP. It can help them understand your sleep issues better and guide any treatment you might need.

Are you sleep deprived?

The answer might be more complex than it first appears, but asking this question is an important starting point. Consider how you spend your days: are you constantly juggling responsibilities, feeling stressed or running on autopilot? How often do you feel tired, foggy, or emotionally drained?

This highlights the classic chicken-and-egg scenario: does a lack of quality sleep create the chaos we feel during the day, or do the chaotic patterns of the day disrupt our ability to sleep? The truth is, it's a bit of both. Poor sleep can amplify stress, make us more emotionally reactive and impair our ability to think clearly. At the same time, an overwhelming or unbalanced day can make it harder to unwind and fall into restful sleep. These two forces feed into each other, creating a cycle that can be hard to break.

While I prefer not to dwell on the scary side of sleep deprivation, it's important to acknowledge that the issue is serious. Poor sleep doesn't just leave you tired; it affects nearly every aspect of health, from cognitive function and mood to immune strength and long-term risks like heart disease and diabetes. But focusing solely on these consequences can feel overwhelming. The more empowering approach is to see sleep as something you can influence – not by trying harder at night, but by reshaping your days.

Am I going to get Alzheimer's if I don't sleep?

This is a question I hear often, and it's completely understandable to be concerned about the relationship between sleep and brain health. As a psychotherapist, I want to first acknowledge that Alzheimer's disease is a highly complex condition, with a wide range of factors contributing to its development, including genetics, lifestyle, environmental influences and, yes, sleep.[12] But the good news is that while sleep plays an important role, a few sleepless nights don't mean you're destined to develop Alzheimer's.

It's worth noting that sleep is essential for brain health in many ways. During deep sleep – particularly slow-wave sleep – the brain's glymphatic system, which acts like a waste disposal network, becomes highly active. This system clears toxins and metabolic waste, including amyloid-beta, a protein linked to Alzheimer's disease. Think of it as the brain's nightly clean-up crew, tidying up the clutter that accumulates during the day.

Some studies have shown that sleep deprivation, even for just one night, can increase amyloid-beta levels in the brain. The US National Institutes of Health, for example, found that a single night of poor sleep can lead to a measurable rise in these levels.[13] But the important thing to remember is that subsequent good sleep can help bring those levels back down. It's not about perfection but about giving your brain consistent opportunities to reset and recover.

The concern arises with chronic sleep deprivation – when poor sleep becomes the norm over months or years. If the glymphatic system doesn't have enough opportunities to clear toxins, it may contribute to the buildup of amyloid plaques over time. But sleep isn't the only factor at play in Alzheimer's. The amyloid hypothesis – the idea that Alzheimer's is primarily caused by amyloid-beta accumulation – has been foundational in research but is also being reexamined, with some scientists suggesting that it's only part of the story.[14] Neurological health is influenced by a complex web of factors, including stress, diet, exercise and mental wellbeing.

So, what does this mean for you? Instead of panicking about the occasional sleepless night, it's more helpful to reflect on what might be behind your sleep struggles. Ask yourself:

- Are you feeling stressed or overwhelmed?
- Could your diet or lack of exercise be affecting your sleep quality?
- Are there underlying health issues, like high blood pressure or depression, contributing to your restless nights?

Tackling these deeper contributors is crucial, as they're often connected to both sleep and overall brain health.

How to work out your true sleep needs

It's best to do this during a holiday when you don't need an alarm clock. It's often on the second week that you start to find where your natural sleep lies. But if you haven't got a holiday coming up, we can still work this out. Use weekends or days off to allow yourself to sleep without an alarm. Track these days separately to compare with your usual sleep schedule. This can give you insight into your natural sleep pattern.

- **Track bedtime:** For two weeks, note the time you naturally go to bed.
- **Track wake time:** For two weeks, record the time you naturally wake up without an alarm or other interruptions.

- **Track sleep quantity:** For two weeks, record the amount of sleep you think you got.
- **Work out your sleep efficiency score:** We tend to look for a sleep efficiency of over 85 per cent to indicate that sleep is going well. By tracking it, you can start to see where improvements are coming. **Important:** This can be stressful for some people so take a view on whether tracking is helpful or not for you.
- **Look for patterns:** Over time, look for consistent patterns in your sleep data. This will help you determine the amount of sleep that leaves you feeling most rested and alert.
- **Experiment:** If it's a regular work week and this is a test-and-learn period, on days when you can afford to sleep more or less, experiment with different amounts of sleep (e.g., seven hours vs eight hours, but don't go too far over this) to see how you feel. Record the results in your sleep diary.
- **Reflect on how you feel:** If you feel well rested with this average sleep duration, it's likely your ideal sleep need.

How to work out your sleep efficiency (%) score

Total time in bed (TIB): Record the total amount of time you spend in bed. This includes all the time from getting into bed to the final waking time in the morning.

Total sleep time (TST): Estimate the total amount of actual sleep you had. This includes all periods of sleep but excludes any time spent awake, such as when trying to fall asleep or after waking up during the night.

Calculate sleep efficiency: Use the formula:

Sleep efficiency (%) =
total sleep time ÷ total time in bed × 100 =
sleep efficiency   %

$$\text{Sleep efficiency}(\%) = \left(\frac{\text{Total sleep time}(\text{TST})}{\text{Total time in bed}(\text{TIB})} \right) \times 100$$

For example, if you spent eight hours in bed (480 minutes) but only slept for seven hours (420 minutes), your sleep efficiency would be: 85.7 per cent

Self-reflection

Things to think about regarding your relationship with sleep and why you might do what you do.

- Am I sleepy (not just tired, but sleepy) by the time I go to bed?
- How do I decide it's time for bed? Is it because I feel sleepy or for some other reason (e.g. it's my habit, because my partner does or because I think I should)?
- How long do I spend in bed each night? Is this very different between weekdays and weekends?
- How long do I spend out of bed each day? How do I spend that time?

Reflect on these questions and consult your sleep diary. How you feel about your sleep might not be accurate. For example, many people believe they wake up at 5 a.m. every day, but it's usually just a memorable coincidence. In truth you might be waking up at varied times and not getting straight out of bed. Keeping a sleep diary builds a tangible picture of your actual sleep patterns – one you can't argue with.

Sleep tech: friend or foe?

Pursuing perfect sleep has catalysed a booming market of gadgets, apps and high-tech mattresses, promising to enhance sleep quality. With the sleep industry projected to grow from $60 billion in 2022 to over $100 billion by 2031,[15] there's a risk that the emphasis on 'wellness' could overshadow proven, evidence-based methods for improving sleep, such as stress reduction, addressing underlying health conditions and acknowledging that sleep is deeply personal – no gadget can fully know 'you' like you do.

Does this sound familiar? You bought a sleep tracker and started fixating on hitting the 'ideal' 85 per cent sleep efficiency. How do you feel on mornings when your tracker shows anything lower? Many people end up feeling anxious, convinced their sleep was poor – even when they actually feel fine. There's a risk of relying on the data to tell you how you 'should' feel, rather than trusting your own body's signals. What started as a tool to improve your sleep can easily become a source of stress instead.

There are so many gadgets to track sleep, from wearables like smart-watches and rings to apps and even 'smart' beds. But, as yet, they tell an incomplete tale. These devices tend to use movement and sometimes heart rate or other physiological signals (like heart rate variability or blood oxygen levels), rather than brain activity, as an indicator of sleep stages, leading to incorrect data. For example, you might be lying on the sofa, scrolling through your phone, but your tracker might wrongly think you're in a light sleep stage – mine does (and yes, I do wear one and have tested many of them, but more for interest than anything else). But the real question is: do you need a device to tell you whether your sleep was restful, or can you trust how your body feels in the morning?

People often tell me that their sleep tracker helps them become more aware of how much sleep they're getting and the timing of it, which can be useful – especially when trying to identify patterns. For example, if you're keeping a sleep diary to track your natural sleep and wake times, the data from a tracker can add helpful context. In these cases, it's best to focus on the consistency of your sleep schedule rather than fixating on the exact amounts of light, deep or REM sleep. It's also worth keeping a flexible attitude about the data.

That said, some trackers offer useful features like real-time oxygen saturation monitoring, which can provide valuable information for your doctor if you're concerned about issues like sleep apnea. Overall, sleep trackers are most effective when used as general guides rather than strict measures of sleep quality.

Ironically, stressing over getting the 'perfect' sleep can make you more anxious and obsessed with every detail. Though not officially recognised as a medical condition, 'orthosomnia' is a term researchers coined in 2017 for this problem.[16] Decoupling someone's stress over their tracker is a common issue in my work. Perhaps the path to true peace lies in keeping it simple, unencumbered by the distractions of technology.

Sleep hygiene – softly, softly . . .

The origin of the term 'sleep hygiene' is not completely clear, but it has been found in an 1864 text by Paolo Mantegazza, an Italian physiologist.[17] I love the observation made by Charles Mercier in his book *Sanity and Insanity* (written in 1890), who offers that 'The way to procure sleep is to observe the hygiene of sleep; to get the body into such a state, and to place it under such conditions and circumstances, that sleep is a natural and inevitable result.'[18] Mercier's observation underscores a timeless truth: sleep should come naturally. But in modern times, as our lifestyles have become more complex, experts like Dr Nathaniel Kleitman and Dr Peter Hauri began to formalise ways to make this natural process easier to achieve. Hauri, in particular, developed practical guidelines for improving sleep in the 1970s, highlighting how what you do before bed – your routines, environment and daily habits – is not mere background noise but directly impacts your sleep quality.[19]

I have a real issue with the term 'sleep hygiene'. It reminds me of 'clean eating', another phrase that carries problematic implications. For me, both terms take fundamental biological processes and wrap them in judgemental language. I especially shudder when I see a headline 'clean up your sleep hygiene!' Like 'clean eating', which implies that there's a 'dirty' way to eat, the term 'sleep hygiene' can create unnecessary pressure. It implies that there's something unsanitary about your natural sleep patterns, adding stress where none should exist.

Sleep hygiene is all about adopting habits that help you sleep better and create a peaceful environment – cool, quiet and calm are the keys. But here's the thing – expecting anyone to suddenly embrace a whole new set of sleep practices overnight is about as realistic as me becoming a concert pianist by next Tuesday.

So, what's the sensible approach? Start by figuring out which sleep habits are most relevant to you. Maybe you're the type who sips espresso after dinner, or perhaps you can't resist one last scroll through social media at midnight. Identify the disruptors based on your own sleep history. Then, tackle them one by one. Make a small change, get comfortable with it, and then move on to the next. It's like climbing a ladder – one rung at a time gets you to the top without the unnecessary risk of a tumble. Improving your sleep needs to be a gentle test-and-learn process, not a wholesale revolution.

The risk is that it becomes a 'thing' – where you might slide into the trap of trying to perfect your pre-sleep routine to the point of absurdity, believing that a specific set of actions is the reason you will sleep rather than trusting that you *can* sleep.[20] It might seem wild, but good sleepers don't do anything to sleep – they just sleep! In our 24/7 media cycle the original simplicity of sleep hygiene has been buried under a mountain of unnecessary advice and clickbait headlines, turning bedtime into a stress-inducing ritual. Suddenly, enjoying a late-night movie or spontaneous plans with friends feels like a crime against your sleep schedule.

Don't forget to keep things simple. Yes, make your bed into the best bed it can be for you. Yes, use earplugs and an eye mask if they work for you (for many people they are essential due to the conditions of their sleep environment). But always remember, sleep, like any natural process, thrives on trust and patience, not micromanagement. So, rather than perfecting your routine, can you focus on what works for you to rest without stress?

Five principles of sleep

I lean into what Professor Colin Espie from the University of Oxford suggests as five simple yet essential principles: to value, prioritise, personalise, trust and protect your sleep.[21] He also emphasises how sleep is personal and different for everyone. I work with people to help them figure out how to make these principles fit into their lives.

Value	To sum up this first principle: value sleep like you would your health. One bad night? No big deal. But long-term, consistent sleep is what supports your wellbeing. The key here is consistency, and it starts with one simple change: set a consistent wake-up time, no matter what. I call this your sleep anchor. Life is unpredictable, especially in the evenings, but a regular wake-up time helps your internal body clock, or circadian rhythm, regulate itself.
Prioritise	Sleep is as essential as brushing your teeth or locking the door before bed – non-negotiable! Listen to your body – if you need to sleep, then sleep. This might mean reshuffling your schedule or letting go of habits that eat into your rest. Your body craves rhythm and routine, so try to maintain regular sleep habits.
Personalise	Understand your unique sleep needs and know your sleep chronotype (see page 110). While seven to nine hours is recommended, this varies for everyone. Get the sleep you need and, if possible, at the time that suits you. Set a consistent wake-up time, even at weekends, and work backwards to determine your bedtime. Stick to this routine for a couple of weeks and see how your body responds. If you're not feeling tired at your designated bedtime, adjust in small increments.

Trust	One of the biggest hurdles to good sleep is trying to control it. But here's the truth: sleep is a natural process. Just like breathing, your body knows how to sleep. If you find yourself lying awake, don't fret but don't lie there rigidly not moving, trying hard to sleep. If you can't sleep after about 15 minutes, get up and do something relaxing until you feel sleepy again.
Protect	Think of sleep as a close friend. Like any important relationship, it thrives on consistency; the more regular your schedule, the easier it will be to stay friends. Don't try to force it – you need to feel sleepy to sleep. Be mindful of what keeps you apart, whether it's stress, screen time or late-night caffeine, and protect your time together. And if you find that your friend sleep is becoming distant, don't hesitate to seek help.

The paradox of sleep effort

The paradox of sleep effort is something Emily knows all too well. A driven, determined person in every aspect of her life – whether in her career, fitness goals or education – Emily approached sleep with the same unyielding focus. But the more she tried, the more elusive sleep became. She had created a rigid pre-sleep routine collated from tips she'd found online, but she often found herself wide awake, staring at the ceiling, her mind buzzing with the irony that the harder she worked at sleep, the further it seemed from her grasp.

It wasn't always like this. There was a time when she could fall asleep as soon as her head hit the pillow. But as life became more demanding, so did her anxiety around sleep. Her resolve to conquer this new challenge only made things worse.

I asked Emily to tell me more about her evenings. She sighed, 'I follow all the advice. No caffeine after lunch, a warm bath before bed and no screens an hour before sleep. I even practise meditation. But the harder I try, the worse it gets. I'm exhausted, but I just can't fall asleep.'

We are firmly in the territory of the paradox of sleep effort; I explain to Emily that sleep isn't something you can achieve through effort.

When you focus too much on sleep, it creates anxiety. Your mind becomes hyper-alert, fixating on the need to sleep, which activates your body's fight-or-flight response, making relaxation – and therefore sleep – nearly impossible. The problem was, she didn't know how to let go.

Meet paradoxical intention – a technique where clients like Emily are encouraged to stay awake rather than trying to sleep. It sounds counterintuitive, but removing the pressure to sleep reduces the anxiety surrounding it.

That night, instead of forcing herself into her lengthy pre-sleep routine, Emily read a book she enjoyed, letting herself become absorbed in the story. I asked her to stop checking her clock and see if she could let go of the need to sleep. I wasn't surprised to get an email from her a couple of days later; she was not impressed – it wasn't working. I advised her to keep going, reminding her not to oversleep the following day and to get up at the same time regardless. To her surprise – and it took three weeks – it worked. It's like reverse psychology for your brain. When you release the relentless pressure to fall asleep, your mind begins to shift gears, creating space for genuine relaxation. This transition allows your nervous system to move out of a state of hyperarousal, and into one of rest and recovery. As the tension subsides, sleep often follows naturally.

If the body knows it's time to sleep, why does sleep disappear when your head hits the pillow?

Once more, the answer lies in how your brain processes the events of the day. Throughout the day, many of us unconsciously suppress or push aside unresolved thoughts and emotions to focus on immediate tasks. But as soon as our head hits the pillow, with no other distractions, these unresolved issues resurface. The brain, now free of external demands, starts processing these thoughts, often triggering the release of cortisol, the stress hormone that ramps up alertness and readiness, which is the exact opposite of what we need for sleep.

This happens because of two key brain systems: the default mode network (DMN), which activates during rest to process lingering worries, and the salience network, which prioritises what's most important. If the DMN is overloaded with worries, the salience network flags them as urgent, keeping your brain in a state of hyperarousal, which makes it hard to sleep.

To help your mind wind down, try setting aside time earlier in the evening to process your thoughts – ideally, right after work. This practice 'offloads' your mental to-do list before bedtime, reducing stress-related brain activity and making it easier to relax and fall asleep. Keep a notebook specifically for this purpose. Set aside ten minutes in the early evening for a worry-time exercise – write down your thoughts, worries or anything else on your mind. After your writing session, review your notes. Highlight actionable problems and cross out theoretical concerns beyond your control. This helps you distinguish between what you can address and what you need to let go of. This practice engages the prefrontal cortex in a controlled way, helping to process these issues before they have the chance to interfere with sleep. Once you've completed the exercise, slam the book shut and tell yourself out loud, 'It's time to let go. I know where the information is, and it's OK to stop trying to solve everything right now.' This reinforces to your brain that it's safe to release these thoughts.

If your bed has become a place for worrying, working or watching TV, your brain starts to associate it with everything but sleep. This is known as conditioned arousal – where the bed triggers wakefulness and anxiety rather than relaxation. That's exactly what had happened to Emily. Emily's issue wasn't that she couldn't sleep – after all, she could easily drift off on the sofa. The real challenge lay in the negative associations she had formed with her bed. While sleeping on the sofa worked temporarily, it eventually backfired, reinforcing her fear of the bed and making her insomnia even worse.

Emily needed a reset – a way to retrain her brain to see her bed as a place for sleep once again. To help her understand, I used her dog, Sami, as an example. I explained that, just as she had trained Sami to pee in a specific spot by rewarding her when she got it right, Emily had once naturally associated her bed with sleep. But if something frightening happened in Sami's usual spot, she'd likely become confused and anxious, just like Emily had with her bed.

So, we took things back to basics. We focused on her sleep from the moment she woke up, establishing a consistent wake-up time and ensuring she got plenty of daylight and movement throughout the day. Regular breaks helped sustain her energy levels, so by evening she wasn't carrying the weight of a stressful day. This created a smoother, more natural transition to sleep. With these foundations in place, we shifted her focus to a relaxed evening routine, freeing her from the pressure of a rigid pre-bed ritual and allowing her to feel genuinely sleepy when it was time to turn in.

This behavioural strategy, often called stimulus control, focuses on reshaping your relationship with sleep and enhancing your sleep environment. By creating a calming bedtime routine and reducing distractions, you can turn bedtime into a truly positive and relaxing experience. This method helps you associate your sleep space with restfulness, paving the way for improved sleep quality. With time and consistency, you'll find that transitioning into sleep becomes easier, leading to a more rejuvenating night's rest and a boost in your overall wellbeing.

To further reduce her anxiety about falling asleep, I introduced Emily to the concept of the sleep window. A sleep window opens when three things align: sleep pressure, your internal body clock and your circadian rhythm. When these elements come together – when you're genuinely tired and your body clock says it's time – you've reached your optimal moment for sleep. If you miss that window, don't worry; another one will usually open in about 45 minutes. So, rather than stressing in bed if sleep doesn't come right away, it's better to get up, do something relaxing and wait for the next window to open.

By combining these strategies and maintaining a consistent wake-up time Emily could retrain her brain to associate the bed with sleep and nothing else.

It's important to remember that this process takes time and consistency. Behavioural changes don't happen overnight, but with patience, Emily broke the cycle of conditioned arousal and started enjoying more restful, restorative sleep.

Do you have to do it all at once?

The question of whether we need one continuous sleep period (monophasic) from approximately 10 p.m. to 6 a.m. remains a topic of ongoing research, particularly when many people work irregular or nontraditional hours. It's also relevant for those whose chronotype – a person's natural sleep–wake pattern – differs from the traditional timing, making it unrealistic for them to conform to a standard sleep schedule.

Understanding sleep from a biopsychosocial perspective provides deep insights into how we rest and how these patterns have evolved over time. Historian Professor Roger Ekirch's research on biphasic sleep offers a fascinating view into historical sleep patterns. Drawing from historical records, Ekirch suggests that people in pre-industrial societies often slept in two phases: a 'first sleep' shortly after dusk, followed by a period of wakefulness known as 'the watch', and then a 'second sleep'. This wakeful period may have been used for reflection, leisure or intimacy, aligning with natural bodily rhythms and environmental cues.[22]

While Ekirch's findings are intriguing, it's important to note that his work is based on historical data rather than modern scientific studies. Imagine if we had the kind of sleep study data from that period that we have today – modern sleep science only truly began in the 20th century, with the invention of EEG technology in the 1920s and 1930s. These early studies laid the groundwork for what we now know as sleep medicine, a field that is still evolving.

Adding another layer of complexity, research from paleoanthropologist Professor Daniel Lieberman suggests that our ancestors likely had more flexible sleep patterns, shaped by environmental conditions such as temperature and social needs, rather than adhering to a strict schedule. This aligns with the idea that before the advent of agriculture and modern society, humans may not have followed a rigid monophasic sleep pattern.

It's possible that what Ekirch describes as 'segmented sleep' might have been a response to natural night-time awakenings due to temperature changes, light exposure or occasional disturbances, rather than a universally practised sleep pattern. The shift towards monophasic sleep, where sleep is condensed into one continuous block, closely correlates with societal changes brought about by the Industrial Revolution. As work hours became standardised, the cultural preference for a single, uninterrupted night's sleep emerged, emphasising productivity and the 9-to-5 workday.

Biologically, this shift makes sense in the context of industrialised work culture, but it doesn't always align with everyone's natural sleep patterns or environment. Sleep isn't a uniform state; it consists of cycles that move through light sleep, deep sleep and REM, with brief awakenings occurring naturally at the end of each cycle. That's why waking up during the night is a normal part of healthy sleep.

That said, there's a difference between normal wakefulness and sleep disruptions that affect your wellbeing. Brief awakenings? Completely normal. But if you're waking up frequently, feeling anxious or struggling to fall back asleep – especially if it's impacting your daily life – it might signal a sleep disorder or another issue that needs addressing. The point isn't to stress about every wake-up, but to recognise when it crosses the threshold into something more concerning.

Making small adjustments to your routine can often lead to better rest. You might feel more energised and better slept by simply shifting your bedtime earlier or later or incorporating a short nap into your day. Some people find that adopting a biphasic sleep pattern – sleeping in two chunks – or aligning their sleep schedule with their natural chronotype, whether you're a night owl or an early bird, makes a noticeable difference.

This flexibility in sleep patterns is further illustrated by how people adjust their sleep during periods like Ramadan, where sleep is naturally segmented due to religious practices. Despite significant changes in eating and sleeping routines, many people maintain their core sleep period at night and top up with a nap during the day, often after the midday prayer, and manage these shifts without major disruptions, underscoring the adaptability of our sleep–wake system.[23]

For those who struggle with waking up in the middle of the night, embracing a segmented sleep pattern could be a more natural and less stressful alternative. But again, there's a line – if it's causing concern or impacting your wellbeing, it's always a good idea to consult a healthcare professional.[24]

A polyphasic sleep approach, where sleep occurs in several segments rather than one continuous block, aligns with the idea that sleep follows natural cycles and can be flexible. However, taking this concept to an extreme brings us to the 'Uberman' sleep schedule. This is the superhuman version of polyphasic sleep, where you take six short naps, each lasting just 20 minutes, spaced evenly throughout the day and night. That totals only about two hours of sleep in a 24-hour period!

The Uberman sleep plan was popularised in the 1990s by Marie Staver, but it's highly unconventional and not without risks. While it's gained attention from those seeking to maximise productivity, this sleep pattern is not recommended for the general population. In fact, studies show that nine out of ten people who tried it had to stop within a month. The one person who managed to continue suffered from symptoms of mania, and their body stopped producing growth hormones.[25]

While some people may thrive on unconventional sleep cycles, the consensus among researchers suggests that monophasic and biphasic sleep patterns are the most conducive to peak cognitive and physical performance.[26] There is no clinical evidence supporting the benefits of extreme polyphasic sleep schedules, and they carry significant risks.

How to experiment with different sleep patterns and timing

Your ideal sleep pattern depends on various factors, including your chronotype, work schedule and lifestyle. Make it personal and work towards finding what works for you. One way to acknowledge your body's unique needs and rhythms is by accepting that a different sleep pattern and timing may suit you better than a monophasic stretch. This acceptance is empowering – you're simply following a path more in tune with your natural needs. I loved the example by writer Joanna Cannon, who found that for her, going to bed at 5 p.m. and getting up just after midnight suits her well and makes life far less stressful.[27] So, I invite you – if you can – to get the amount of sleep you need at the time that suits you. And if you're a couple, prioritise your individual sleep needs. If that means sleeping separately, so be it – better rest for both of you can lead to a healthier, stronger relationship.

First, we look at your sleep diary to see your current habits (see page 46). Next, we decide on a wake-up time that fits your schedule – like when you need to be at work. Then, we work backwards from your wake-up time to figure out the best time for you to go to bed. It can take a few weeks to get this timing embedded, especially if we are working on getting you to align the timing seven days a week.[28]

Why would you want a regular sleep/wake time?

The brain and body thrive on rhythm, so keeping your bedtime and wake time consistent supports your natural circadian cycles. This is often the first thing we address when reviewing a sleep diary, as irregular sleep patterns can disrupt these rhythms, putting your body in a state similar to chronic jet lag. In this state, getting the rest you need becomes much harder.

By going to bed and waking up at the same time every day, you establish a routine that your internal clock can rely on. The body loves predictability – it learns when it's time to sleep and when it's time to wake, making the whole process smoother and more restorative. Avoid falling into a cycle of sleepless nights followed by oversleeping; this feast-or-famine approach throws off your rhythm and leaves you feeling out of sync.

Waking up at a consistent time also helps your body align with natural light, which sets your internal clock for the day. Regular morning light exposure can improve digestion, boost alertness and enhance overall wellbeing. Don't underestimate the power of consistency – especially when it comes to waking up at the same time each day. It's one of the most effective ways to improve your sleep quality.

Anchor sleep

Anchor sleep is the core period of sleep that most of us experience in the first half of the night. In sleep patterns, particularly when exploring polyphasic sleep schedules, anchor sleep is the primary pillar of rest. This core period is complemented by additional, shorter naps sprinkled throughout the day. Three key points to anchor your sleep:

- **Consistency:** The same sleep period is maintained daily, even on days off.
- **Core sleep:** This is the most important part of the sleep cycle, often occurring during the night or early morning.

- **Flexibility:** Additional sleep periods can be added, but the timing of the anchor sleep remains consistent.

Imagine anchor sleep as the steady heartbeat of your nightly routine. It's that one unwavering stretch of sleep you prioritise at the same time each night, offering your body a dependable rhythm. This consistency helps to regulate your circadian rhythms, the internal clockwork that governs so much of your biological functioning.

For those who navigate the challenging waters of shift work, it becomes a lifeline if you can anchor your sleep. It gives a robust synchronisation of your biological rhythms, improving overall sleep quality and cognitive performance.

Predictability in our ever-changing lives can be hard won, but anything you can do at the same time every day – including mealtimes and when you go to the loo for a number two, your body will thank you for. It can be challenging at first, but as it becomes habitual, the stress of creating a new routine will disappear as your internal and external worlds line up as they should.

How to RISE UP: A morning routine to improve your sleep

When you're struggling with sleep, finding the energy to work on strategies can feel overwhelming – especially when you're already exhausted. That's why this book encourages you to tackle your sleep issues at moments that are low-pressure, rather than focusing on the stress of bedtime or those sleepless hours in the middle of the night. Instead, shift your attention to when you wake up. Though it might feel counterintuitive to get out of bed instead of trying to squeeze in a few more minutes of rest, dedicating time at the start of your day is one of the most effective ways to build habits that can improve your sleep in the long run.

Dr Allison Harvey's RISE-UP routine offers a powerful framework for this. Here's how to incorporate her approach into your morning to set yourself up for better sleep:[29]

- **R: Rise at the same time each day**
  Aim to wake up at a consistent time every day, even at weekends. This helps regulate your body's internal clock.
- **I: Immediately get out of bed**
  Resist the temptation to hit snooze. Getting up as soon as you wake helps signal to your body that it's time to start the day.
- **S: Start moving**
  Engage in some light physical activity, whether it's stretching, a short walk or a few exercises. Movement boosts your energy levels and helps shake off morning grogginess.
- **E: Expose yourself to light**
  Get as much natural light as possible in the morning. Light exposure sets your circadian rhythm and improves alertness throughout the day. I am keen on daylight alarm clocks too, to help build this light exposure.
- **U: Upbeat music**
  Energise your mood with music that lifts your spirits.
- **P: Protein-based breakfast**
  Avoid the sugar spikes from a sugary breakfast. Fuel your body with a protein-based breakfast to keep you sustained and focused.
- **Make a to-do list:** Set your intentions for the day. Organising your tasks can reduce anxiety and help you feel more in control.
- **Check in with yourself:** Take a few deep breaths and assess how you're feeling. A moment of mindfulness can set a positive tone for the day.
- **Take a morning walk:** If you're working from home, mimic the effect of a commute by going for a brief walk. This can help transition your mind into work mode and provide a natural break between waking up and starting your workday.

Why more sleep won't solve the tiredness

If you have insomnia, you might think spending more time in bed would help, but this can make things worse. It can lead to lighter, less restful sleep. Instead, spending less time in bed can be more effective. As we saw with Emily, sleep restriction therapy (SRT), or consolidation, helps to concentrate your sleep and improve its quality.

Just as trying to stay in bed longer to 'catch up' on sleep often back-fires, the same goes for trying to catch up at weekends. The idea that you can compensate for sleep lost during the week by sleeping longer at weekends is a misconception. Chronic sleep debt can't be repaid in one or two nights of extended sleep. To recover, prioritise consistent rest and gradually add 15–30 minutes of sleep each night to restore what's been lost.

It's logical to think that more sleep should equal more recovery, right? But here's where the data surprises us: regularly sleeping more than nine hours a night can be just as problematic as not getting enough.

When oversleeping becomes a habit, the consequences are less rosy. Research tells us that consistently oversleeping is associated with higher risks of lethargy, cognitive sluggishness, and even chronic conditions like diabetes, heart disease and obesity. And here's the sobering truth: it's also linked to higher mortality rates.

So why isn't more sleep the universal cure we think it is? Assuming that sleeping more will fix the problem is logical when you're tired. But that's like pouring water into a bucket with a hole in the bottom – it doesn't address the deeper issue. Sleep quality trumps sleep quantity every time. It's not about how many hours you log in bed; it's about how effectively you move through the crucial stages of sleep – light, deep and REM. The idea of the 'perfect' eight hours? That's a myth we need to leave behind. Your body needs the right amount of sleep tailored to you – sometimes, less than eight hours, but with better quality.

Let go of the obsession with hitting a magic number of hours. The goal isn't checking off an eight-hour box; it's waking up feeling restored, even if you've had fewer hours than what's often discussed. Can you stop counting hours and instead focus on how you feel?

You might also wonder, 'Can I save up sleep and use it later?' The concept is seductive – like a hack for busy people. Sleep a few extra hours at the weekend and magically create a reserve of energy for the week ahead. Unfortunately, it doesn't work that way. Sleep isn't something you can hoard or stockpile like holiday days. Our bodies, intricate and dynamic, resist such simple solutions.

Pre-emptive napping, on the other hand, does have its merits – but only in specific circumstances. A planned nap can relieve fatigue and improve focus for shift workers or anyone with an unpredictable schedule. Research shows that a well-timed nap can reduce cognitive wear and tear, enhance alertness and restore some of the energy you'll need to power through. If you know a period of disrupted sleep is coming – like a night shift or a long travel schedule – a nap beforehand can help.

But here's the caveat: it's not a long-term solution. It's a patch, not a repair.

The allure of pre-emptive sleep reflects a deeper yearning: the desire to master our biology and outwit the natural rhythms that govern it. But no matter how clever we think we are, the body isn't easily tricked. Our internal clocks need regularity, not sporadic fixes. They crave consistency – the key is living life at a rhythm that allows for deep, restorative sleep night after night.

Think of how you feel after staying up late at the weekend and dragging yourself out of bed for work on Monday. It's that groggy, out-of-sync feeling, as if you've crossed a time zone without leaving your house. Sleeping in to 'catch up' only disrupts your natural rhythm further, creating a vicious cycle that leaves you more exhausted than before. While it may seem like a quick fix, those extra weekend hours can do more harm than good in the long run.

An unfortunate truth remains: irregular sleep patterns disrupt our circadian rhythm. Our biological time and societal time often seem to operate on entirely different clocks. While society has divided life into neat, precise units – hours, days, years – our bodies follow rhythms that are far less rigid and predictable. Social schedules, like work and school, often clash with our natural sleep preferences, which is especially true for night owls, who have a significant mismatch between their sleep schedules on workdays and weekends. This mismatch leads to a phenomenon that chronobiologist Professor Till Roenneberg calls 'social jetlag',[30] where our bodies are perpetually out of sync with the expectations of the world around us. This mismatch can lead to sleep deprivation, making you feel tired and less alert. It affects your metabolism and overall energy levels, disrupting how your body regulates hunger and fullness, which can lead to unhealthy eating patterns, weight gain and further strain on your system.[31]

Sleep is not something to hoard, ration or hack. It's a daily practice, a relationship with your body that you need to nurture, one night at a time.

So, if more sleep isn't going to improve how you are feeling, what is? We need to think seriously about rest – taking breaks when we need to. It is not a luxury or a waste of time.

You need real, profound rest. The kind that rejuvenates both body and soul.

Think of the difference between holding yourself upright with effort and control, versus letting go completely – every muscle relaxing and letting go of tension. Both are beneficial, but only one provides that deep, undisturbed rest that your entire being craves. Real rest is about dialling out, allowing your entire being to reset and rejuvenate. Getting more of it during your waking hours is key, and we'll explore this concept in more detail in the chapters that follow.

Summary

Too often, falling asleep feels like a frustrating task, but it doesn't have to be. With the right mindset, it can become something to look forward to – a time to relax, reflect and unwind. Even if you're not falling asleep right away, simply being in bed to rest has its own value. Resting gives your mind and body a chance to reset, recharge and prepare for the day ahead. Sleep may be the goal, but rest is never wasted.

Beyond the basics, this chapter explores how falling asleep is a gradual, natural process. One highlight is the hypnagogic state – the dreamy transition between wakefulness and sleep. This magical space, where creativity stirs and thoughts flow freely, isn't just a step towards rest – it's an experience to savour.

Along the way, you might encounter normal sleep phenomena, like hypnic jerks (those sudden jolts), sleep inertia (morning grogginess) or even sleep paralysis. These are not failures, but natural quirks of the sleep process. Understanding them can ease your anxiety and make the journey to sleep feel less intimidating.

We also dipped into the world of lucid dreaming, where you can become aware of and even influence your dreams. This fascinating state can spark creativity or offer therapeutic benefits, such as helping process trauma or confront fears in a safe, dreamlike space.

Falling asleep isn't something to conquer; it's a chance to let go. And even on nights when sleep feels elusive, resting in bed can still bring comfort, healing and peace. By embracing the value of rest and sleep alike, you can transform bedtime into a soothing, even enjoyable, experience.

Actionable steps

- A good night's sleep starts when you wake up. Incorporate the RISE UP routine to set a positive tone for the day.
- Protect sleep. See it as a friend, not something to fear or hate.
- Keep a sleep diary to track your sleep patterns and identify potential circadian rhythm misalignments.
  - Establish a baseline for how much sleep you need.
  - Set a consistent wake-up time, even at weekends.
- Allow your mind to wander as you relax in bed, paying attention to the images and sensations that arise naturally.
- Keep a notebook by your bed to jot down creative or intriguing thoughts. It won't disrupt you falling asleep – it should help.
- When it comes to sleep, we are looking for quality, not quantity. It's better to have six hours of deep, restful sleep than eight hours of tossing and turning.
- If sleep doesn't come, don't force it. Get out of bed, do something relaxing and return to bed when you feel sleepy again.

- Track your sleep patterns, stressors and daily activities but don't obsess to identify what impacts your sleep.
- Set aside time earlier in the evening for a 'worry dump' to offload unresolved thoughts and reduce bedtime stress.
- True rest isn't only about sleep. Make time for mental and emotional relaxation during the day to help your body and mind unwind, making it easier to sleep well at night.

CHAPTER THREE

Connecting the dots: how sleep responds to life

Driving down the motorway, I'm often struck by the hidden lives around me. Every vehicle carries someone with a unique story, their own web of thoughts, yet we all share this common journey. Life mirrors this road – individual paths briefly intersecting, our actions subtly influencing one another in ways we rarely acknowledge. Just as the flow of traffic is shaped by countless decisions, small and large, sleep is similarly governed by the seemingly minor details of our daily existence – our routines, thoughts and the stressors we carry. These ripples, often imperceptible, accumulate and shape how we rest and sleep, reflecting the deeper interplay between body and mind.

Meet Alex, a 38-year-old father of two, who had recently started experiencing restless nights. Alex used to be an avid runner, finding solace and clarity during his early morning jogs. These runs weren't just about staying fit – they were a time for him to clear his mind, connect with his thoughts and prepare himself for the day ahead. After his runs, he would sit down with his family for breakfast, sharing stories and enjoying those few quiet moments before the hustle of the day began. But as his job grew more demanding and the responsibilities of parenthood increased, those morning runs became less frequent, eventually disappearing altogether.

Alex's sleep issues weren't just about stress or poor routines; they were part of a larger picture that included the loss of his regular running habit – a physical outlet that had once helped him manage stress. Without the mental clarity his runs provided, he found himself carrying the weight of his stress throughout the day. His mind, once calm and clear from the steady rhythm of running, now felt cluttered and overwhelmed. Morning family breakfasts, once a comforting ritual of connection, had dwindled as well, replaced by rushed meals or skipped altogether in the scramble to get everyone out the door. These gradual shifts chipped away at Alex's ability to unwind, ultimately making it harder for him to get restful sleep at night.

Many of us find that our routines – whether it's exercise, family time or simply taking a moment to breathe – are often the first things to go when life gets busy. Yet, these routines matter for our wellbeing. They provide structure, help us manage stress and create a sense of normality in our lives. When we lose touch with them, it can disrupt our mental and physical health, leading to issues like insomnia.

When I asked Alex, 'What do you need to support yourself right now?' it wasn't just about managing stress – it was about rediscovering the routines that once gave him stability. Alex decided to bring running back into his life, just a short jog a few times a week to begin with. He also committed to having breakfast with his family at least three mornings a week, creating a simple ritual that set a positive tone for the day. These small yet meaningful changes helped him feel more centred, and in turn, his sleep began to improve.

So, as you consider your own sleep, perhaps it's time to reconnect with a part of your daily routine that's been neglected – whether it's regular exercise, family time or simply taking a moment each day for yourself. Sometimes the solutions seem obvious, but it's easy to lose sight of what matters most in life's busyness. Talking it through with a trusted friend, loved one or therapist can provide the perspective and support you need to refocus your habits.

The big picture

When working with clients, I might work through a visual process with them using a process based on the biopsychosocial (BPS) model, developed by psychiatrist George Engel.[1] Unlike the traditional biomedical model, which focuses solely on physical ailments, the BPS model looks at the bigger picture. It highlights how your lived experiences, emotional states and bodily processes interact, helping shed light on the 'strange logic' of sleeplessness and its root causes. I bring out pens and paper, and we physically map out how each aspect intertwines to affect sleep, health and wellbeing.

It can be an unexpectedly powerful process. It tends to get us both out of our chairs, moving around and seeing things from different angles. It slows down the conversation, encouraging reflection, and allows space to identify connections not made before. For example, as we will see, you might suddenly realise that a late-night work routine isn't just a habit – it's tied to feelings of guilt about not 'doing enough' during the day.

Creating your own biopsychosocial map is a reflective and insightful process, helping you to understand the diverse factors influencing your thoughts, behaviours and wellbeing. Here's a simplified guide to get you started:

Creating your own biopsychosocial map

- Find a large piece of paper – an off-cut of wallpaper is perfect for this. Also a variety of coloured pens or markers.
- Draw the core circles: start by drawing three large circles on your paper, each representing one of the core factors of the biopsychosocial model: Biological, Psychological and Social.
- From each circle, draw branches that represent different aspects or subcategories within each core factor. For instance:
  - Biological: branches could include genetics, physical health, sleep patterns or neurological factors.
  - Psychological: branches here might represent emotional health, coping strategies, personal beliefs or past trauma.
  - Social: this circle's branches includes areas like family dynamics, cultural background, social interactions or work environment.
- Use different colours to highlight or categorise the branches. This not only makes your map visually appealing but also helps in organising your thoughts.

- Within each branch, jot down specific elements that are relevant to you. For instance, under the 'Biological' circle, you might write about any chronic illnesses or your typical sleep patterns.

As you map out these details, reflect on how these factors interconnect and influence each other. For example, how does your work environment (Social) affect your stress levels (Psychological), and in turn, how does that influence your sleep quality (Biological)?

Look for patterns or areas that might need attention or improvement. This could be a stressor in your social circle impacting your psychological wellbeing or a biological factor affecting your social interactions.

Remember, your biopsychosocial map is not static. It's a living document that can change as your circumstances or understanding evolve.

This mapping process is a creative and personal endeavour. There's no right or wrong way to do it – it's about exploring and understanding your own unique life situation.

This hands-on approach transforms the process into something collaborative and grounded. Instead of just talking *about* sleep issues, we work together to uncover patterns, make connections and create a roadmap for meaningful change.

Working with Zina, a 43-year-old parent, illustrates how this process works. The social aspects of her life – balancing job insecurity, parenting and endless responsibilities – are having a physiological and psychological impact: she is emotionally and physically drained.

At work, Zina feels constant pressure to prove her worth. Working in a company where she is the only person who is a parent, her situation is often glossed over. Evenings offer little relief – her mind races, replaying the events of the day and catastrophising about what lies ahead. This stress triggers a late-night 'second wind', driven by elevated cortisol levels, which keeps her awake and working until midnight or later.

Her sleep diary reveals a deeper, more nuanced issue: Zina isn't giving herself enough time in bed to get the sleep she needs. This comes back to the BPS loop – biologically, her elevated cortisol levels make it difficult for her body to settle into sleep, but psychologically, her reactive mindset compounds the problem. Instead of allowing herself to lie quietly during periods of wakefulness – when sleep might still be possible – she reacts immediately by getting out of bed and overriding her body's chance to rest. This pattern reinforces the idea that sleep is futile, further disrupting her natural sleep–wake cycle and training her body to expect wakefulness in the early hours of the morning, preventing her from getting the full spectrum of sleep stages, including REM sleep, which is needed for emotional regulation and memory consolidation.

'When I wake up, I'm wide awake,' she told me. 'It's like sleep has completely disappeared. So, why waste time trying to force it? I just get up and work before switching into parent mode.'

Instead of getting up at 4 a.m., could she experiment with staying in bed to give her body the chance to recalibrate? Even light sleep or quiet rest has value – it reinforces the body's natural rhythm and provides opportunities for restorative sleep to return.

There's a tricky balance to managing this situation. If stress or anxiety creeps in while lying awake, engaging in a calm, non-stimulating activity like reading, listening to a podcast or journalling can prevent the bed from becoming associated with frustration but if anxiety really spikes, then it's time to get out of bed and do something else. If you cannot get back to sleep – remember, the longer you are awake, the likelihood is that the next time your body will take the recovery it needs to compensate.

How to map out your 24 hours to review where you spend your energy

Purpose: Understand how you spend your day and make sure you have enough time for your basic needs.

What you'll need: Pen and paper, or a digital tool (like a spreadsheet or time tracking app).

Time required: 24 hours of tracking + 30–60 minutes for review and planning.

Create a pie chart or table to represent each hour of the day.

Make categories: Sleep, Nutrition, Hygiene, Physical activity, Work/Study, Leisure, Other.

For one full day, jot down what you do each hour. Be detailed and mark activities that take up multiple hours.

Remember to prioritise your basic needs, such as eating regularly, staying hydrated and taking necessary toilet breaks.

Think in terms of:

Sleep: Aim for 7–9 hours.

Nutrition: Plan for three to five meals, whatever works for you, 30–60 minutes each (including prep time).

Hygiene: Spend 30–60 minutes on personal care.

Physical activity: Get at least 30 minutes of movement.

Reflect on this – it can be surprising!

Review your time log at the end of the day.

Ask yourself:

- Did I get enough sleep, nutrition, hygiene, and exercise?
- Were there activities that took more time than expected?
- Did I spend time on things that matter to me?

Plan and adjust:

Based on your reflections, adjust your schedule.

Make sure to set aside time for your basic needs first, then fit in other activities.

Put it into practice:

- Follow your new schedule.
- Be flexible and adjust as needed but try to stick to the basics.

Helpful tips:

- Be honest when tracking your time.

- Use alarms or reminders to help you transition between activities.
- The goal is to find a structure that supports your wellbeing and productivity.

Reflection points:
- Are you eating and drinking enough?
- Are you getting enough sleep?
- Are your social interactions fulfilling?
- Is screen time affecting other activities?
- How do different environments impact you?
- Are there patterns in your stress levels?

Next steps:
- Identify 1–3 areas you'd like to improve.
- List specific actions to make these changes.
- Set a timeline to implement these changes.

Check-in: Revisit this exercise now and then to make sure you're still on track with your wellbeing goals.

Reminder: Every day is unique. Use this exercise as a guide, and adapt it as needed for your wellbeing.

Psychological factors and mental load

Many people, like Zina, fall into the trap of thinking, *'I have too much to do – sleep can wait.'* It seems logical: if you're behind on tasks, you should keep working to catch up. But this is a fallacy. You can't 'bank' or 'catch up' on missed sleep later. Sleep is critical for both physical and mental functioning, and without it, productivity and wellbeing suffer.

During sleep, particularly REM sleep, the brain processes and integrates new information, consolidating it from short-term to long-term memory. Cutting sleep short disrupts this process, making it harder to retain new information and recall it later. A well-rested brain, on the other hand, is more efficient, creative and capable of solving problems effectively. Sleep isn't wasted time – it's the fuel that powers your ability to handle tasks more quickly and with better focus.[2]

> ## Going without sleep can make you as impaired as being drunk. Here's a simple breakdown:
>
> Being awake for **17–19 hours** slows thinking and reaction times, akin to having a blood alcohol content (BAC) of **0.05 per cent**.
>
> Staying awake for **24 hours** is even worse, equivalent to a BAC of **0.10 per cent**, which is over the legal driving limit.
>
> Both sleep deprivation and alcohol impair your coordination, decision-making, and response time. A lecture I once attended illustrated this with a powerful example: accidents caused by either sleep deprivation or alcohol often show no skid marks. Why? Because the impairment prevents the driver from reacting in time. Similarly, when you're sleep-deprived, you make poor decisions, act impulsively and struggle to manage emotional responses – just as if you were tipsy.

In another session we examined the psychological factors and mental load contributing to Zina's sleep issue – the stress of the impact of mental load. Mental load refers to the invisible, ongoing effort of managing and organising the many responsibilities and tasks in your life. It's not just about completing tasks – it's about constantly *thinking* about them, planning, remembering and anticipating what needs to be done. For instance, it's not just packing a child's bag for school; it's remembering that it's swimming day, checking if the goggles are in the bag, realising sunscreen needs to be restocked and making a mental note to pick some up later – all while balancing work deadlines, family schedules and household chores.

Mental load wreaks havoc with sleep and stress because it keeps the brain's hypothalamic-pituitary-adrenal (HPA) axis activated. This system regulates the release of cortisol, the body's primary stress hormone, which in turn suppresses melatonin release, delaying the body's ability to feel sleepy. It also activates the amygdala, the brain's emotional processing centre, overriding the prefrontal cortex's ability to apply rational thought or emotional regulation.

I ask Zina to describe her evening thought process when deciding whether to go to bed. At first, she said she doesn't even think about it, but after pausing, she corrected herself:

'No, that's not true. I know I need to sleep, but there's this over-whelming sense of responsibility. I start thinking about all the things I haven't finished and everything I need to do tomorrow. And then these negative thoughts just keep coming. I can't seem to unwind.'

Zina's response revealed a pattern of anticipatory anxiety and rumination – her mind is so focused on unfinished tasks and future worries that she struggles to relax. But beneath this lies a deeper question: Why is she driving herself so hard?

When I explored this with her, Zina admitted feeling like she was failing in every area of her life – at work, as a parent and even in taking care of herself. This sense of inadequacy was fuelling her emotional arousal, intensifying her stress and worsening her sleep problems.

As we continued working through Zina's situation, the social aspect of her mental load began to emerge. I noticed she rarely mentioned her partner in our sessions, so I asked how they handle stress together and whether she feels supported in the relationship.

Her response was telling: 'We don't talk much now. We don't have time.'

Zina and her partner live far from friends and family, which limits their access to external support. At work, she feels isolated as the only working parent, and at home, she perceives an unequal distribution of domestic responsibilities. These social dynamics leave her feeling like everything rests solely on her shoulders, adding to her mental and emotional load.

It's true that certain aspects of Zina's situation, such as living far from friends and family, would take time to address, and some challenges are not easily solved. However, by using the biopsychosocial model and mapping out how she spends her time, we were able to create a clear plan of action. While it's impossible to fix everything at once, breaking her situation into smaller, manageable parts allowed us to identify patterns, prioritise her most pressing needs and begin building healthier habits step by step.

Importantly, by helping Zina improve her sleep, we could shift her outlook. When better rested, her brain would be less prone to negativity and overwhelm, and the bigger picture might not feel quite so insurmountable. Zina's situation is all too common but examining your life in this way can reveal areas that need attention that might otherwise sit below the surface.

It's been a rough day

Sometimes, unhealthy coping mechanisms feel impossible to resist. When healthier options don't seem to be working, it's OK to choose what feels manageable and causes the least harm. Ordering takeout, pouring a glass of wine or binge-watching Netflix can be comforting, releasing dopamine and helping you unwind. No judgement here – it's a normal way to relax after a long day.

But does it truly help you recharge and sleep? Staying up late for 'just one more episode' can leave you groggy the next day, and alcohol or heavy meals close to bedtime can disrupt your sleep cycle. While comforting in the moment, these habits fall into the category of passive relaxation – a temporary escape that doesn't fully address the underlying stress or emotions.

Then there's the question of what happens to the stress and emotions you've carried all day. Do they fade away, or are they simply paused – waiting to resurface in the form of rumination when the distractions wear off? Coping through passive relaxation, like binge-watching or drinking, often silences feelings temporarily, but those unresolved thoughts can rush back just as your brain is trying to rest.

Instead of viewing relaxation as a choice between 'right' or 'wrong' behaviours, it's about exploring what genuinely nourishes you. Passive relaxation has its place – it's OK to indulge in Netflix, takeout or a small glass of wine – but pairing these with intentional, active relaxation can make all the difference. True relaxation goes beyond comfort or distraction. It involves calming your nervous system and allowing your body to shift from a stressed, 'fight-or-flight' state (sympathetic nervous system) into the parasympathetic 'rest-and-digest' mode. This state reduces cortisol, aids digestion, and prepares your mind and body for rest. Not only does this help you unwind more deeply, but it also clears the way for better sleep, allowing you to wake up feeling more rested and recharged.

I often use the analogy of a fizzy drink bottle: each stressor shakes the bottle a little more, increasing internal pressure. By the end of the day, trying to sleep is like opening an over-shaken bottle – it's messy, leaving you wide awake.

This accumulated pressure doesn't just disrupt the ability to fall asleep; it causes early morning awakenings and affects mood, causing irritation and a tendency to adopt coping strategies like sugar or alcohol. The body's 'alarm system' stays stuck in the 'on' position, keeping you in a constant state of high alert.

The solution isn't complex routines but simple, manageable interventions to 'release the fizz' throughout the day. This could be a short meditation, a walk outside or deep breathing – small acts that gradually relieve stress and prevent it from building to a night-time peak. By pacing stress management across the day, you can shift from a cycle of exhaustion to a more peaceful, natural sleep pattern.

When rumination is the issue

One of the biggest obstacles to sleep is rumination – when your mind gets stuck on a problem, replaying it over and over, often right when you're trying to wind down for the night. Rumination often masquerades as problem-solving, tricking us into believing that if we think hard enough, we'll find clarity. Yet, like Zina, many find themselves digging deeper into anxiety and catastrophic thinking instead of solutions. It's a common thread I've seen in my work – this fixation on negative content that keeps us anchored to our distress.

Psychologists have long studied rumination, exploring its different facets. There's brooding, where we dwell on our problems without seeking resolution, and there's reflective pondering, which can lead to insights if guided constructively. The challenge lies in recognising when introspection turns into a detrimental loop.[3]

But rumination doesn't stop at affecting our emotions; it reaches into our physical wellbeing too. Recent studies have shown that persistent negative thinking can amplify physical pain and hinder recovery. Our minds and bodies are more connected than we often acknowledge. When the mind is in turmoil, the body frequently responds in kind.

Do you often find yourself lying in bed, wide awake, with your mind suddenly springing back to a problem at work or a challenge you faced earlier in the day? This is a classic case of rumination – your brain thinks that it is trying to help you but it's going to keep you awake.

The prefrontal cortex, responsible for complex thinking and decision-making, becomes highly active during rumination. It's working over-time, trying to solve a problem by analysing it from every angle. However, this intense focus on the problem is powered by the stress response, which is a product of how our brain predicts and constructs emotional experiences based on past learning.

During rumination, the brain's attempt to be helpful can backfire, especially when you're trying to sleep. The brain predicts that by going over a problem repeatedly, it will find a solution. However, this continuous loop keeps the brain in a state of high alert, making it difficult to transition into sleep.

At the same time, the amygdala, the part of the brain that deals with emotion, tags these repetitive thoughts as significant or even threatening. When the amygdala flags these thoughts, it's as if your brain is predicting that these concerns are important and require immediate attention. This emotional tagging intensifies your feelings, reinforcing the brain's prediction that these thoughts are urgent – and keeping you wide awake.

When you notice your mind slipping into rumination, the first step is to deliberately pause and take a deep breath. This simple act can help disrupt the brain's predictive loop by momentarily calming the stress response. Breathing deeply activates the parasympathetic nervous system, which counteracts the stress response, allowing the prefrontal cortex – the part of your brain responsible for complex thinking and decision-making – to reset. By regularly practising this mindful inter-ruption, you can begin to regain control over your thoughts, preventing them from spiralling out of control just as you're trying to sleep.

If the rumination is worry-induced, there's another approach that aligns with how the brain functions. Instead of trying to deny or suppress the worry, which can often intensify the cycle, you can acknowledge the worry, understand its purpose and then consciously direct it elsewhere. This approach is based on the understanding that your brain is trying to help by bringing these concerns to your attention. It's spinning these thoughts round and round in an effort to solve a problem or avoid a perceived threat.

By acknowledging the worry, you validate the brain's predictive process – essentially telling your brain, 'I see you're trying to help, and I appreciate that.' From here, rather than letting the worry take over, you can practise 'taming' it by consciously boxing it up in a mental 'container' or allowing yourself a controlled time to worry. These techniques leverage your brain's natural tendency to categorise and organise information, allowing you to feel more in control.

How to box up those issues

This is similar to the worry-time exercise (see page 58) but uses a different learning style for those for whom the thought of writing for ten minutes is off-putting. It's a simple way to control when and where you deal with your worries and can be done at any time of the day.

- You need: a small box (like a shoebox), paper and pen, a timer or alarm.
- Think about what's bothering you. It could be stress, a worry or a problem that's taking up too much of your energy.
- Write or draw the issue on a piece of paper. Just naming the problem can help you start to deal with it.
- Fold the paper and put it in the box. As you close the lid, say out loud, 'I am in control of when I choose to engage with this' (or words to that effect – make it yours, even if you express yourself in other ways).
- Choose specific times each day to focus on the issue. For example, ten minutes in the morning and evening. Use a timer for these periods.

- When you feel able, find a quiet spot, open the box and take out the paper. Spend the designated time thinking or working on the issue. Focus fully, knowing you'll put it away when the time is up.
- When the timer goes off, stop. Fold the paper, put it back in the box and close the lid. Make a conscious effort to think about other things until the next scheduled time.
- At the end of the week, think about how this process went. Did it help you manage the issue? Were you more productive or less anxious at other times?

By using this 'worry box', you can contain your stress and manage it in a controlled way, freeing up your mind for other activities.

Are you angry?

Anger or its stronger cousin, rage, can be a tricky subject. There seems to be a certain taboo to admitting feelings of either and yet both are valid. Instead, they get bottled up, repressed, buried, but have a habit of appearing when you aren't expecting it, with a tendency to do damage. It's also very hard to sleep if you are angry.

Picture this: you're navigating a busy day, balancing life's countless demands, when suddenly a minor annoyance sets you off. You pause and wonder, *'Am I more irritable than I used to be?'* or perhaps even, *'Why does everyone around me seem angrier these days?'* If this sounds familiar, you're not alone. Growing clinical evidence suggests that our modern lifestyles may indeed be contributing to a rise in anger – and no, it's not just down to poor sleep and social media.

Our diet has undergone significant changes in recent decades, with a sharp rise in the consumption of ultra-processed foods. One emerging theory for the increase in anger and emotional dysregulation links this dietary shift to the gut microbiome – the complex ecosystem of trillions of tiny organisms living in our digestive system. These microbes play a key role in digestion, immune function and mood regulation through the gut–brain axis. When our diet is poor, the balance of the microbiome can be disrupted, leading to the production of toxins and systemic inflammation. This inflammation can affect brain function, influencing mood and behaviours like irritability and anger.[4]

Now, imagine the relentless heat of a scorching summer's day. It's not just uncomfortable; it's a stressor that can exacerbate irritability and aggression and keep you awake. Researchers have noted that with the ongoing climate crisis, we are increasingly exposed to conditions that elevate stress and anger. The hotter it gets, the more we tend to find ourselves on edge, ready to snap at the slightest provocation.[5]

Adding to this is the economic and social climate. Picture the high stakes of modern life: competitive job markets, skyrocketing living costs and the pressure to keep up with social expectations. These factors create a zero-sum game where the competition for resources and opportunities is fierce. This environment breeds frustration and anger when things don't go as planned, amplifying feelings of helplessness and rage.[6]

Overlay this with the broader mental health landscape. Anger is not just a standalone emotion; it's often a symptom of deeper psychological distress. Conditions like depression, anxiety and PTSD have become more prevalent, partly due to the stresses of modern living and global uncertainties. Research has shown how the pandemic has left many feeling isolated and anxious, further contributing to a general rise in anger.[7]

In this swirling mix of gut health, environmental stress, economic pressures and mental health challenges, we become quick to anger and stuck in states of aggression and defence. But there's hope. Understanding these underlying factors gives us the power to address them. For instance, improving our diet, finding ways to manage stress and seeking support for mental health issues can help mitigate these feelings of anger.

So, next time you feel a wave of anger rising, take a moment to consider the broader picture. What are you really trying to express?

To further explore how anger and unaddressed emotions can wreak havoc on sleep, let's meet Frances. In her 40s, Frances juggles a demanding career in insurance, a family and the invisible weight of unexpressed anger. Her story sheds light on the deeper psychological battles that contribute to insomnia.

In her first session, Frances shares that she doesn't want to be seeing me, that I can't help her, that her insomnia is untreatable. Her challenge to me is explicit – almost telling me this is going to fail before we start. She pushes her sleep diary towards me, a thick, worn notebook filled with meticulous records of restless nights.

I gently tell her that right now I'm not interested in her sleep diary, instead asking, if she thinks I can't help her, why has she come in? (This highlights a point that sometimes sleep diaries are helpful and some-times they aren't. It depends on your relationship to it.)

Her eyes flash with a mix of defiance and desperation. 'Because . . . I don't know what else to do,' she admits, 'I'm exhausted and . . . raging. All the time. And I don't know why.' It could be, like Zina, that sleep deprivation and stress are playing a part, but the intransigence of her insomnia makes me wonder. I ask if she can tell me about the rage.

Frances shifts uncomfortably in her chair, crossing her arms tightly over her chest. 'It's just . . . everything. Work is a nightmare, my husband is clueless, and the kids . . . God, the kids. I love them, but they drive me insane. And now, my body is betraying me too. I'm 46 and peri-menopausal, and it feels like everything is spiralling out of control.'

Biologically, being peri-menopausal introduces a layer of complexity, particularly due to fluctuations in progesterone and oestrogen levels, which also have a direct impact on sleep. Progesterone, which has a natural calming and sedative effect, declines earlier and more sharply than oestrogen during this stage. This can lead to difficulty falling or staying asleep, as the brain loses this soothing influence on the nervous system. Meanwhile, fluctuating oestrogen levels further disrupt sleep by affecting the regulation of serotonin and melatonin – two key hormones involved in maintaining a healthy sleep–wake cycle.

These hormonal changes can also trigger night sweats and hot flushes, which fragment sleep and leave the body feeling more stressed and depleted. Poor sleep, in turn, lowers the brain's ability to regulate emotions and manage stress, creating a vicious cycle where sleep depriv-ation amplifies the emotional effects of hormonal imbalances.

When Frances described feeling rage, it became clear that this wasn't simply a reaction to external stressors. The combination of lower progesterone (which normally calms the nervous system), erratic oestrogen (which influences emotional sensitivity) and disrupted sleep sets the stage for heightened irritability and emotional outbursts. Rage, in this context, can feel overwhelming because the brain and body are struggling to regulate both emotional and physical stressors simultaneously. But with Frances I am curious. Rage feels bigger, hotter than anger – what is fuelling her rage?

Frances looks at me, her eyes dark and stormy. 'I don't know,' she whispers. 'I feel like there's this . . . this volcano inside me. I've kept it bottled up for so long, trying to be the perfect wife, be the perfect weight, the perfect mother, the perfect employee. But it's getting harder and harder to contain it. And the insomnia . . . it just makes everything worse. I can't keep doing this.' As she speaks, I can see the pain and frustration etched on her face.

It sounds like there's a lot more going on here than just trouble sleeping. Her referral also mentions bruxism – teeth grinding or jaw clenching that can happen both when you are awake or asleep – and migraines, and she has seen a neurologist and had scans to rule out anything significant. I notice her hand unconsciously rubbing her jaw, a sign of her bruxism, and I ask her about it. 'I can't seem to stop grinding my teeth. My dentist says it's stress.'

It's fascinating how the body can reflect what the mind is struggling to process. In Frances's case, the immense tension she carries seems to speak volumes. Suppressing what she's feeling might be contributing to her jaw clenching in a cycle of teeth-grinding resentment and frustration, with migraines and bruxism potentially acting as physical manifestations of this bottled-up anger.

Of course, I recognise that there could also be a medical explanation for her symptoms, such as hormonal changes, muscle tension or even a neurological condition. But my interest lies in exploring the psychological dimension – how emotions we struggle to express or even acknowledge can translate into physical pain. So, I ask her gently, *'What do you think you might be trying to hold back?'*

She considers this, her eyes filling with tears she quickly blinks away. 'I don't know. Maybe everything. The frustration with my job, my husband, the kids . . . the feeling that I'm failing at everything. Maybe I'm just trying to keep it all together?'

It's a lot and I share with her that it's no wonder her body is reacting this way. Insomnia is a logical response because repressed anger keeps the body stuck in a state of stress and hypervigilance, both of which are incompatible with the calm and restorative state required for sleep.

Releasing the anger

So, what can you do with anger when it builds up in your body? The urge to move, to scream or to lash out is a natural response – these are your body's way of trying to release pent-up emotions but for many reasons they just aren't possible or appropriate. Imagine anger like throwing a punch but stopping midway. The unspent force, the unresolved emotion, stays trapped inside, creating tension that can manifest as insomnia, anxiety or physical discomfort.

Dr Peter Levine, the psychologist and developer of somatic experiencing (SE),[8] and a pioneer in trauma therapy, often uses the example of an impala on the savannah to illustrate how animals naturally process stress. Imagine watching a wildlife documentary: an impala grazes peacefully, fully relaxed. Suddenly, a lion begins stalking it. The impala's nervous system snaps to attention, preparing for flight. Once the impala escapes, it instinctively shakes from head to tail, discharging the adrenaline and resetting its nervous system. This process allows it to release the trauma of the chase and return to a calm state.

We humans, however, often disrupt this natural process. Instead of shaking off traumatic energy, we might suppress our physiological responses, leading to stored trauma that can manifest as anger. How, then, do we complete these natural responses? By finding safe spaces where the body can release pent-up energy and return to equilibrium, much like the impala shaking off its brush with death.

It's a deeply human concern, and while the research is extensive, consensus remains elusive. Take primal scream therapy, for instance. Developed by Arthur Janov in the 1970s, this technique has shown some success. Participants often report feeling emotionally lighter and less burdened after expressing their anger through a primal scream. It's a raw, visceral release that some of my clients find useful – I've suggested they climb a hill and scream into the open air, or even scream into the water while swimming. These actions can offer temporary relief but they often fail to address the deeper underlying issues causing the anger; for some people they are even distinctly unhelpful. Rage and anger don't appear out of nowhere; they are signals, pointing towards unresolved emotional turmoil that demands our attention. Like the bottle of fizzy drink, we need to let off the pressure bit by bit.

Levine suggests that traumatic experiences and intense emotions, such as anger, can become 'stuck' if they aren't processed effectively.[9] From a neurobiological perspective, this makes sense – trauma triggers the sympathetic nervous system, raising norepinephrine levels. This hormone promotes alertness and vigilance, which can lead to difficulty falling asleep and staying asleep.

I often recommend bodywork techniques, either with a practitioner, or through activities like boxing, aikido or jiu-jitsu with instructors who understand the value of channelling anger and rage constructively. These practices provide a structured environment where the body can learn how to complete its natural fight-or-flight responses, which, in the past, may have been blocked or thwarted.

My focus with Frances is on helping her work with her anger – finding ways to acknowledge and move through it, while providing immediate strategies to release some of that built-up tension so she can finally let go.

I see her nodding, albeit hesitantly. It's clear that she's been overwhelmed by the insistence on finding a concrete reason for her insomnia.

I explain that this may be why her sleep diary doesn't hold the answers, and that there is a chance that the keeping of such a long-term record might be part of what's fuelling her insomnia.

Frances looks puzzled. 'How so?'

A sleep diary can be a helpful tool for uncovering patterns and identifying sleep issues, allowing you to connect the dots and make changes to improve your rest. For some, it offers valuable insights and those 'aha!' moments. However, constantly monitoring and recording your sleep patterns can create a sense of hyper-awareness and anxiety about sleep. Every night becomes a test *you're* afraid of failing. This stress about not sleeping can make it harder to sleep. The diary turns sleep into a task rather than a natural process, which can be counter-productive.

So, instead of focusing on how well or poorly she is sleeping, I ask if we can target the underlying psychological rage and release some of that pent-up energy first.

Frances took up boxing sessions at the gym and found that combined with journalling to process emotions, she'd discovered a channel to release her rage. This shift reduced her tension and eased her insomnia.

Try things that genuinely lift your spirits and really feel them. Call up a friend, go to a football match with your mates, sing in a choir or dive into a hobby you love. Change your physical state to change your mental state.

For many people, movement is more effective than stillness when it comes to managing emotions like anger or fear. Physical activity helps release built-up tension and repressed feelings while improving mood and reducing stress.

Find what makes you feel good and focus on that. Everyone's different, and it's about discovering what helps you personally. Don't stress about what doesn't work – treat it as an adventure, trying new things until you find what hits the spot.

Time to put the brakes on

In a world that values constant productivity, slowing down might seem counterintuitive. Still, research shows it can reduce overwhelm and improve productivity, mental health and overall quality of life.[10] When you slow down and become mindful, you can become present. Presence gives you the space to see where you really are in that moment and what you need to do next rather than everything all at once. It's about diving deep rather than skimming the surface.

Come back to ground

A simple grounding exercise to help you feel more present starts with focusing on your feet. Take a few deep breaths. Notice how your feet feel on the ground and wiggle your toes. Then, look around and wiggle your fingers. This shifts your attention to the edges of your body, reminding you that you are more than just your core organs. This practice can help activate the rest-and-digest response, promoting calm and relaxation.

Becoming mindful

Mindfulness is an ancient practice that has spanned thousands of years. It is a way of paying attention that can be practised formally (through meditation) and informally (in daily activities). Professor John Kabat-Zinn defines it as 'awareness that arises through paying attention, on purpose, in the present moment, non-judgementally'.[11] It offers the potential to come into the here and now, to be with your thoughts, emotions, bodily sensations and actions without self-judgement or criticism. It's not about zoning out; it's about accepting whatever you are experiencing in the present moment without striving for a particular state of mind.

It offers a gentle way to calm the nervous system and reduce stress, naturally enhancing sleep quality. By being present and slowing down, you can sustain steady energy levels and align with your natural rhythms, enabling you to notice and appreciate small moments often missed in the rush of life. While society pushes us to move faster, slowing down can significantly reduce stress, anxiety and the risk of burnout. Some people find it challenging, but it's not advisable for all and there are other ways to calm the nervous system through movement and exercise.[12] But if it works for you, then it's all good. Research shows that mindfulness can help prevent depression, reduce anxiety, ease chronic pain, control binge-eating and help you stay calm and relaxed in difficult situations.[13]

While it's true that no one is 100 per cent mindful all the time, the more you practice mindfulness, the more control you gain over your life. It allows you to slow down, think before you act, and question that pervasive negativity bias – are things *really* as bad as they seem?

Are you feeling sleepy or tired, or are you just overwhelmed?

Tired, you might catch yourself drifting off during the day – your head nodding at your desk or your eyes drooping in front of the TV. Irritability might creep in, but a solid night's sleep is usually enough to reset your mood and energy. However, if you're severely sleep-deprived, the need for rest can feel far more intense, and the consequences go beyond mere drowsiness. Long-term sleep loss can lead to concentration problems, memory lapses and poor work performance. Irritability can linger, straining your relationships and making daily interactions more challenging.

Take a moment to check in with yourself (a moment of mindfulness). What emotions or thoughts are coming up for you right now? Can you acknowledge these internal experiences without judgement? Now, shift your attention to your body. Notice any physical sensations – tension, fatigue, discomfort, or perhaps even hints of relaxation or sleepiness? These sensations can provide valuable clues about your body's needs.

For instance, ongoing fatigue might signal more than just a lack of sleep; it could be a sign of overwhelming stress – but it is also a classic symptom of sleep apnea. Recognising the difference is essential, as treating sleep issues without addressing underlying stress won't resolve the root problem. Sleep gets the blame for a lot of things – you might believe you're tired because you didn't get enough of it, but there are almost infinite reasons why you might be tired:

- Lack of daytime light exposure
- Overwhelm
- Feeling unsafe
- Too much time online
- Stress and anxiety
- Hormonal changes
- Parenting at any age
- Being a carer
- Working in an open-plan office (see page 194)
- Substance use, including nicotine, caffeine, sugar and cannabis
- Lack of movement

Research into thinking styles has revealed that people with more severe insomnia tend to dwell more on their fatigue, often thinking about how tired they feel and how they lack the energy to get through the day.[14] They may also hold unhelpful beliefs about sleep or self-diagnose as insomniacs. But if a lack of sleep causes fatigue, sleeping more should make the tiredness disappear, right?

Not quite. The relationship between sleep and fatigue is tricky. Studies show that even when people with insomnia receive treatment and their sleep improves, they often still feel tired during the day. One study found that students with insomnia who were treated for their sleep issues experienced better sleep but still felt fatigued. Another study discovered that therapy for insomnia doesn't always alleviate daytime fatigue, indicating that improving sleep alone might not be sufficient to resolve feelings of tiredness, suggesting other underlying things contribute to fatigue in those with insomnia.[15]

When you focus on something, it signals to your brain that it's important. This is like the 'pink elephant paradox': if I tell you about a pink elephant and then say not to think about it, you'll find it hard to avoid thinking about it. This paradox shows how our focus can affect attention, especially regarding sleep.

While focusing on something is natural, becoming preoccupied with it can start to increase stress. When you fixate on sleep, your brain interprets it as being highly important, which can elevate stress levels. This stress and anxiety strengthen the neural pathways associated with these emotions, creating a cycle where worrying about sleep makes it even harder to achieve.

This anxiety disrupts your sleep patterns, turning into a self-fulfilling prophecy. The more you stress about sleep, the harder it becomes to fall asleep. This aligns with psychologist Daniel Wegner's ironic process theory[16] (instead of pink elephants, he used white bears), which rather than suppressing or directing specific thoughts or feelings, we inadvertently amplify them, making insomnia worse.

This cycle shows how a mindset focused on fatigue and negative sleep beliefs can exacerbate feelings of tiredness and further disrupt sleep, illustrating the impact of thoughts on our physical state.

Positive perspective in three, two, one . . .

Three steps to quickly reframe a negative thought into a positive one:

- **Step 1: Spot the negative thought**
  Start by noticing what's really bothering you about your sleep. ,
  Example: *'I keep waking up in the middle of the night, and it's ruining my sleep.'*
- **Step 2: Gently reframe it**
  Instead of getting stuck in frustration, try softening the thought with a more even perspective.
  Example: *'Yes, I'm waking up, but it doesn't mean the whole night is ruined. I can still find rest in the time I have.'*
- **Step 3: Focus on what you can do**
  Now, shift your attention to small, calming actions that help you feel in control.
  Example: *'When I wake up, I can try a few deep breaths or a relaxing stretch, rather than stressing about the clock.'*

By the end of this quick exercise, you've transformed a negative thought into a source of motivation in just three steps. This can be done anytime you need a quick mindset shift.

I think of anxiety reduction as finding ways to turn the heat down or let the pressure out of the bottle of fizzy drink. Little by little, lots of small actions do precisely that. Becoming more mindful of how you are feeling can help you to differentiate between whether you are tired or sleepy. Accepting that stress happens will allow you to experience it without added guilt or pressure. This acceptance can help you discover ways to manage it, such as seeking support, prioritising your wellbeing and being kind to yourself. Remember, acknowledging your stress is a healthy step towards managing it better.

How to manage daytime tiredness	
Things that increase the risk of stress and poor sleep	*Positive steps to reduce stress and improve sleep*
• Falling into negative thought traps • Cancelling plans due to fatigue leads to isolation (e.g., skipping the gym or social activities) • Obsessing over whether you will get a good night's sleep • Trying to do everything due to unrealistic self-expectations increases mental load • Using adrenaline to continue working	• Notice and challenge negative thoughts and question whether they're true. • Have meetings with colleagues outside the office, either in a coffee shop or while walking. • Share the burden of life's minutiae with trusted others. • Take regular breaks to shake your body out and breathe.

Crashing out

'Crashing out' describes the sudden onset of extreme sleepiness, often after a period of prolonged sleep deprivation or chronic exhaustion. It's the equivalent of a phone battery dropping to 1 per cent with no warning, and it leaves you barely able to keep your eyes open. This can lead to microsleeps – brief moments where the brain slips into sleep mode, even while you're still 'awake' – which can be dangerous, particularly when driving or operating machinery. These microsleeps can last a few seconds to minutes, making reaction times and decision-making as bad as being drunk. Sleep disorders like sleep apnea make these risks even worse. Major accidents, such as the Bhopal gas leak and the Three Mile Island and Chernobyl nuclear disasters, have been linked to performance failures due to lack of sleep.[17] Temporary fixes like caffeine, fresh air or loud music are ineffective and dangerous, as they don't address the body's need for rest and may increase risks, particularly in high-vigilance professions.

Signs to watch for

• When you're nearing a 'crash', you may notice yourself yawning frequently or feeling a sense of physical heaviness, especially in the eyelids.

- You might find that your mind is drifting, or that you're staring blankly without fully processing what's in front of you. This is an early sign that your brain is entering microsleep mode.
- Difficulty concentrating or remembering what you were just doing or thinking about can be a sign that your brain is exhausted and struggling to keep up.
- If you catch yourself blinking longer than normal or feel your head nodding, it's a sign that your body is struggling to stay awake.

Caffeine

Lots of people rely on caffeine – the world's favourite pick-me-up – to stay awake and fight off tiredness. It works by blocking adenosine receptors in the brain. Adenosine is a chemical that builds up throughout the day, creating 'sleep pressure' – the feeling that it's time to rest (remember, previously, we compared this to saving up sleepy coins to spend on sleep). By blocking this process, caffeine delays those drowsy feelings temporarily. It also triggers the release of adrenaline and dopamine, giving you a boost in focus and mood.

But here's the catch: caffeine doesn't stop adenosine from being produced; it just holds it off for a while. When the caffeine wears off, adenosine rushes back in, often causing a rebound effect – what we know as a major energy crash. This can leave you feeling worse than before and often craving more caffeine to compensate, which can increase the risk of dependence.

What's interesting is that our response to caffeine varies widely due to genetics. Some people metabolise caffeine quickly and feel energised and focused, while others process it more slowly and might feel jittery or anxious. Research shows that genetic differences in how we break down caffeine and how sensitive our brain's receptors are to it can make a huge difference in how caffeine affects each of us.[18]

Recent studies also indicate potential health benefits of caffeine, particularly for neurodegenerative diseases like Parkinson's and

Huntington's.[19] However, caffeine's sleep-disrupting effects are often more pronounced in older adults.[20]

As people age, their metabolism slows, including the activity of CYP1A2,[21] the liver enzyme responsible for breaking down caffeine. This slower metabolism means caffeine stays in the body longer, increasing the risk of prolonged wakefulness and reduced sleep quality.

Ageing also brings natural changes to sleep architecture. Older adults spend less time in deep, restorative sleep and often experience more fragmented sleep. Caffeine, which blocks the sleep-promoting effects of adenosine, can worsen these age-related sleep disruptions, making it harder to achieve restful sleep. Additionally, age-related shifts in circadian rhythm often lead to earlier bedtimes and wake-up times. Caffeine, especially when consumed later in the day, can interfere with these rhythms, delaying sleep onset and further disturbing the natural sleep cycle.

Interestingly, caffeine may have a calming effect on individuals with ADHD, a phenomenon related to how caffeine interacts with the brain's dopamine system. Dopamine is a neurotransmitter involved in pleasure, attention and movement, and people with ADHD often have dysregulated dopamine levels. By increasing dopamine, caffeine can help reduce hyperactivity and improve focus, producing a calming effect rather than the jitteriness it might cause in others.[22] This reaction is similar to the effects of stimulant medications used to treat ADHD, though caffeine is not a substitute for prescribed medication.

Mindful caffeine

I'm not against caffeine, just mindful of timing and quantity. If you love coffee or tea, turn your morning cup into a mindful ritual. Serve it in a beautiful mug and take a moment to sit and truly savour it. This simple enjoyment of your morning caffeine can be a wonderful way to reduce stress and start your day on a positive note.

But if you're out and about, it can be challenging to know just how much caffeine you are consuming. Research conducted by the UK consumer advocacy organisation Which? uncovered substantial differences in caffeine levels from various high-street coffee shops, with some containing up to six times more caffeine than others.[23]

To better manage your intake, it's a good idea to ask about the type of beans and brewing methods used. Being mindful of serving sizes and potentially opting for smaller or weaker drinks can also help you keep your caffeine consumption within your desired limits.

The problem with the increasing use of energy drinks among teenagers

You might have noticed more teenagers consuming energy drinks, and this trend is worrying due to the potential health risks. In the UK, political parties are considering banning these drinks for under-16s – this is not a 'nanny state' action, it's common sense. The issue lies in how children's bodies handle these drinks differently from adults. A 13-year-old boy, weighing half as much as an adult, feels the effects of caffeine much more intensely.[24] Despite clear health risks the high caffeine content is particularly problematic for younger individuals, disrupting their already changing sleep patterns and possibly increasing risky behaviours.[25] Energy drinks are popular due to viral marketing and celebrity endorsements, making them appealing to teenagers, who often feel invincible and may not fully understand the harmful effects of excessive caffeine.

Are nootropics worth it?

The idea of using substances to enhance cognitive function dates back thousands of years, with natural nootropics like ginseng, caffeine and herbal remedies being used in traditional medicine across cultures.

I'm often asked about all kinds of strategies and solutions for staying awake or getting to sleep – some of which, admittedly, can seem a little questionable.

As a psychotherapist, I'm not medically trained, but I make it a priority to stay informed about the substances and techniques people are exploring. By understanding what's out there, I can meet my clients where they are, provide informed support, and weave this knowledge into therapy in a way that's both compassionate and effective.

The modern term 'nootropics' was coined in the 1970s by Corneliu Giurgea, a Romanian chemist and psychologist, who described them as substances that improve brain function, memory and learning with minimal side effects.

What's new today is the mainstream rebranding and marketing of nootropics, fuelled by the wellness industry and the tech world's obsession with productivity and biohacking. Advances in neuroscience and consumer demand have expanded the range of products, blending ancient remedies with cutting-edge synthetics. As a result, nootropics are now presented as tools not just for addressing cognitive decline but also for optimising peak mental performance. Their exponential rise in popularity really hit me when watching the popular series *Clarkson's Farm* with their (hilarious alien invasion) adventures in growing lion's mane mushrooms.[26]

Lion's mane (*Hericium erinaceus*) mushroom has been used in traditional Chinese medicine for centuries, and modern research has started to validate some of its cognitive-enhancing properties, but as yet much of the research on lion's mane has been conducted in animal models or small human trials. Larger, more comprehensive studies are needed to fully understand its efficacy and safety.

Others, like *Ginkgo biloba* and ginseng, have been used for centuries, but the evidence for these herbs is mixed. Caffeine we know about, and L-theanine, an amino acid found in tea, is said to promote a state of relaxed alertness.

What are we really chasing? While pills, potions and supplements promise the magic of sharper focus and endless energy, the most effective tools are often the simplest – sunlight on your face, movement in your body, nourishing food and restful sleep. Yet, these aren't the quick fixes we've been conditioned to crave.

The real question isn't about alertness – it's about expectation. Our culture worships productivity, demanding we operate at full capacity every moment of the day. But this relentless drive ignores something essential: our energy isn't a straight line; it ebbs and flows, just like everything else in life.

What would happen if we stopped chasing endless output and instead turned our attention inward, asking, *What do I really need right now?* Maybe it's not another jolt of energy, but permission to pause, breathe and be. True performance isn't found in the endless push; it's in learning to work with the natural rhythm of who you are.

The influence of diet on sleep quality

It's widely accepted that avoiding heavy, sugary or overly spiced meals before bed – and limiting caffeine and alcohol – can improve sleep. But this advice often feels like addressing the symptoms of a deeper issue.

We live in an era full of contradictions when it comes to food. On one hand, satisfying a craving has never been easier – just a few taps on a smartphone, and dinner is at your doorstep. Yet, for many, the convenience of this accessibility comes at a cost. If your diet leans heavily on foods high in fat, sugar and salt while leaving out fruits, vegetables, fibre and lean proteins, the impact on your health can feel inevitable. But for so many people, this isn't a matter of choice – it's a reflection of the relentless demands of modern life.

Time has become a precious resource, and preparing a meal from scratch can sometimes feel less like an option and more like an impossible luxury. And even for those who want to make healthier choices, the reality of where they live can often limit what's possible in the growing number of communities referred to as 'food deserts', where shelf-stable goods dominate and affordable, fresh, and nutritious food is painfully scarce.

What also concerns me is not just what we eat but why. The psychology of our relationship with food is central – not just to physical health but to how we perceive ourselves and, by extension, how we sleep. Sleep, after all, is not simply a physiological state. It's a barometer of inner harmony, influenced by biological rhythms and the stories we tell ourselves about our choices.

Food, sleep and the modern crisis

As a psychotherapist, I frequently work with clients grappling with the psychological weight of their dietary habits. Many feel trapped between contradictory nutritional or dietary advice and the overwhelming lure of hyper-palatable engineered foods. These foods are far from neutral;

they are scientifically designed to override satiety, hijacking the brain's reward systems.

Obesity, in particular, lies at the heart of this crisis. It is not merely a matter of willpower or individual failing but a complex web of genetics, neurobiology, psychology and the pervasive influence of modern food systems. Its ripple effects touch every dimension of health, including sleep, where the impact is significant. Studies show that approximately 70 per cent of individuals with obesity experience obstructive sleep apnea (OSA),[27] leading to fragmented, poor-quality rest and chronic fatigue. Fragmented sleep, drops in oxygen levels and nights spent in a state of chronic stress are common. Beyond the clinical markers, I often witness a significant emotional cost: the experience of feeling trapped in a cycle – battling cravings and systemic forces that feel insurmountable.

Ultra-processed foods: hysteria or healthy concern

The role of ultra-processed foods (UPFs) in this crisis has become a focal point of public health discourse. Studies link UPFs to a host of metabolic issues – diabetes, hypertension, dyslipidemia (too much fat in the blood) and, of course, obesity[28] – all of which exacerbate sleep problems. This attention has raised awareness but also led to unintended consequences. The term 'UPFs' encompasses a broad spectrum of foods that are not all created equal. Probiotic yoghurt is considered ultra-processed, but so is a bag of crisps. Where would we be without infant formula milk? For some, the push to eliminate UPFs fuels perfection-ism and disordered eating patterns, compounding psychological stress. In addition, research into the impact of UPFs on our health is still ongoing, leaving the public adrift amid conflicting messages.[29]

I work with clients in therapy to explore and disentangle their feelings about these narratives. Food choices should feel empowering, not paralysing, and it's essential to approach diet with a mindset of balance, curiosity and self-compassion – rather than fear or perfectionism.

The role of hormones: leptin, ghrelin and sleep

The link between sleep deprivation and dietary choices is another key piece of the puzzle. Sleep loss – less than five hours a night on an ongoing basis – inverts leptin and ghrelin, the hormones that regulate hunger and satiety. A meta-analysis of observational studies reviewed data from over 600,000 adults and found that individuals sleeping less than five hours per night were at a 55 per cent increased risk of developing obesity compared with those sleeping seven to eight hours per night. Hormonal disruptions, particularly in leptin and ghrelin, were identified as key mechanisms driving this relationship.[30]

Leptin, often called the 'satiety hormone', signals to the brain that you've had enough to eat. When you're well rested, leptin levels are sufficient to keep this feedback loop intact. But when sleep is restricted, leptin levels drop, dulling the brain's ability to recognise fullness.

At the same time, ghrelin, the 'hunger hormone', is elevated during sleep deprivation. Produced in the stomach, ghrelin stimulates appetite, essentially shouting at the brain, 'You're starving!' The result is a double whammy: low leptin whispers, 'You're not full,' while high ghrelin screams, 'Feed me!'

One study found that getting only four hours of sleep per night for just two nights caused hormonal changes that made people 24 per cent hungrier, especially craving calorie-packed, carb-heavy foods.[31] Research consistently shows that sleep-deprived individuals are drawn to sugary, fatty and salty options – the hyper-palatable, ultra-processed foods that dominate today's food environment. Worse, sleep deprivation also impairs the prefrontal cortex, the brain region responsible for impulse control and decision-making. This combination of heightened cravings and reduced self-control creates a perfect storm for overeating.

Over time therefore, chronic sleep deprivation drives weight gain, metabolic dysfunction and an increased risk of obesity, diabetes and cardiovascular disease – all of which, in turn, further disrupt sleep. It's a self-perpetuating loop.

Breaking this cycle is not about willpower – the narratives of blame and moral failing oversimplify a deeply complex issue. Reducing obesity, improving sleep and fostering better relationships with food cannot be solved by gritting your teeth and 'just trying harder'. They require a compassionate understanding of the many forces at play: biological, psychological, environmental and systemic. So, when clients come to me with obesity-related sleep issues, it's not my role to look at *what* they're eating – that is the job of a dietician. Instead, I explore *why* and *how*. Food is never just food. It's a reflection of time scarcity, industrialised systems, cultural messaging and the narratives we all internalise about control, pleasure, shame and worth.

This is one of the reasons why many of my medical colleagues who work in this space are excited about the potential of GLP-1 receptor agonist drugs, such as semaglutide. These drugs, such as Ozempic and Wegovy, which regulate appetite and blood sugar levels, can offer an additional tool to support individuals in breaking out of the relentless cycles of hunger and overconsumption. Importantly, though, drugs like these are not magic bullets, and there are side effects so you should always consult a healthcare professional. They also cannot replace the foundational work of building healthier sleep habits, addressing the psychological aspects of food relationships and confronting the broader systemic issues that make healthy living so tricky for many people.

Alcohol and sleeping pills as sleep aids

The quest for restful sleep can lead people down the well-trodden paths of alcohol consumption and the use of over-the-counter remedies or prescription sleeping pills. In the UK, where drinking culture is deeply ingrained, many turn to alcohol as a seemingly quick fix for sleepless nights. Surveys indicate that about 20–30 per cent of people report using alcohol as a sleep aid occasionally, with higher usage seen in older adults and those suffering from sleep disorders.[32]

The science gives us a clear warning. Drinking more than one standard drink for women or two for men within three hours of bedtime can really mess up your sleep. Even a lunchtime drink can affect sleep. Alcohol is metabolised at approximately one unit per hour, so depending on how much you consume, its effects could still be present by bedtime, subtly impacting your body's ability to settle into restorative sleep.

Here in the UK, a standard drink is a 330ml beer, a 175ml glass of wine or a 25ml shot of spirits. While alcohol might help you fall asleep faster, especially when you're stressed, anxious or dealing with insomnia, its effects are misleading. It starts as a sedative but often leads to broken sleep, frequent wake-ups (including trips to the loo) and less REM sleep. This broken, poor-quality sleep can actually make the stress and anxiety you're trying to avoid even worse.

In my practice, I often see people who enjoy a drink or two – or three – and wonder where the line is between a harmless habit and a problem. It's a difficult one to answer. Enjoying a drink can be a part of socialising or unwinding after a long day, and that's perfectly normal, but it depends on so many variables, how much, how often, what you are drinking and so on. It's also a cultural norm, which can make it a hard habit to break.

If you're having a couple of drinks occasionally and it doesn't interfere with your sleep, health or daily life, then it might not be an issue. However, it's important to be honest with yourself about why you're drinking and how it affects you. When drinking becomes a regular way to cope with stress or emotions, or if you find yourself needing more to get the same effect, it could be a sign of a developing problem.

For those who snore or have sleep apnea, alcohol will make it worse. It relaxes the muscles in your throat, making the airway more likely to collapse and cause breathing problems while you sleep. So, while a nightcap might seem like an excellent way to wind down, it's not doing your sleep any favours. Cutting back on alcohol, especially right before bed, can help you get better, more restful sleep. Equally, understanding the impact alcohol has means you can choose to accept its consequences instead of blaming sleep. Similarly, while sleeping pills have their place and can offer short-term relief, they come with their own set of risks. Dependency, cognitive impairment and even increased mortality rates are associated with long-term use of these medications. They are, at best, a temporary solution and not without significant trade-offs.

Self-reflection exercise

Accepting the consequences of drinking means moving away from a judgement-oriented mindset and towards a more introspective one. This shift requires a conscious effort to observe and understand your body's responses. How does alcohol influence your sleep quality? Do you notice increased anxiety or irritability after a night of drinking? Are there patterns in your behaviour or thought processes that emerge after alcohol consumption?

By exploring these questions, you can begin to make more informed choices about your drinking habits. This doesn't necessarily mean abstinence, but rather a mindful approach to consumption. It's about recognising that the short-term pleasure of a drink might come with long-term costs and deciding whether those costs are worth it.

When snoring indicates a far more significant issue

While it's easy to brush off snoring as just a noisy annoyance, it can sometimes be a sign of something more serious. It can be a signal that your body is struggling during sleep, potentially due to obstructed airways or other issues. If your snoring is frequent, loud or accompanied by other symptoms like daytime fatigue, it's important to take it seriously and consider seeking medical advice to rule out conditions like sleep apnea (see Chapter Seven for more on the different types of apnea disorders).

It can also trigger insomnia in your bed partner, who can often report dreading going to bed due to your snoring, putting strain on both health and relationships, even risking a 'sleep divorce' where couples sleep separately to ensure better rest. This is not necessarily a 'bad' thing; better slept, your relationship is likely to improve.

Summary

Mindfulness and slowing down are not mere trends but vital practices that can profoundly affect our health and happiness. By paying attention to your sleep signals and finding moments of relaxation throughout the day, you can better align with your natural rhythms and improve quality of life.

Societal pressures and factors that influence behaviour, from an everything everywhere all at once culture to the glorification of busyness, call for a broader understanding and a compassionate approach. Recognising the interconnectedness of our actions and their impacts can foster a more empathetic and supportive environment for everyone.

Ultimately, we must connect the dots between our lived experiences and bodily responses to foster a holistic approach to health. By acknowledging the interdependence of our psychological, social and biological systems, we can create more effective and compassionate strategies for wellbeing, allowing us to navigate the complexities of life with greater ease and understanding.

Actionable steps

- Understand how your daily interactions and actions impact your sleep. Write down how different parts of your day make you feel.
- Identify what disrupts your sleep. It might be obvious, like a partner's snoring, or it might be a little more unrecognised, like resentment about unequally shared family responsibilities. Use solutions such as earplugs and regularly reviewing the status quo.
- Regularly ask yourself, 'What do I need to feel supported right now?' Write down your answers and take steps to meet those needs.
- Use the biopsychosocial (BPS) model to see how your thoughts, social life and health affect your sleep. Map these out and find ways to improve them.
- Are there deeper issues that might cause stress and keep you awake? This could mean seeing a therapist or practising mindfulness and stress management techniques.
- Check how your relationships impact your sleep. Improve communication, seek support from friends and family, and consider couples therapy if needed.
- Stay mindful of that second wind. Exercise, get some sunlight and take short breaks to help you feel sleepy at night.

- Know that rest is different from sleep. Take regular breaks during the day to reduce stress levels.
- Keep an eye on diet and weight – consult a dietician or nutritionist if you need help.
- Remember to keep things in perspective. Some nights are good, some nights are bad, but overall, the body knows how to sleep.

CHAPTER FOUR

Master the rhythm of time

Despite the undeniably negative impact of the pandemic on many people's sleep and mental health, about a quarter of those who previously had insomnia experienced significant improvements in their sleep during this period, which contrasts with the experiences of those who were good sleepers before the pandemic, some of whom saw their sleep quality get worse.[1] One study highlighted how people tended to sleep longer and start their day later during lockdown weekdays, reflecting a move towards more flexible and consistent sleep schedules.[2] An end to commuting and packed weekends led to a less hectic life for many. Others have mentioned feeling like they had more time. So, what changed?

With the move to working from home, commuting stopped, and with fewer social obligations, many of us felt a slower, more relaxed rhythm to daily life, which brought better sleep to some previously plagued by insomnia. With the chance to sleep in line with their natural rhythms rather than a rigid schedule, many experienced better rest and reduced stress. This slower pace gave some of us a sense of having more time – and more control over our schedules.

This newfound extra time was channelled into restful or new activities at home. Lego building became hugely popular[3] as did baking sourdough bread. Baking bread requires time, and during the pandemic, baking sourdough peaked on social media, perhaps reflecting a retreat to the home where time suddenly opened new possibilities.[4] So, while the hours didn't change, how we experienced them highlighted how much lifestyle impacts sleep and wellbeing.

Tick tock, body clock

Time may be a social construct, but your biological clock has its own rules. Some people are wired to go to bed at 9 p.m., others at 3 a.m.– all guided by their unique circadian rhythms.

The body's natural timers of cellular, molecular and biological activities repeat roughly every 24 hours. Controlled by an internal 'master clock' in the brain's suprachiasmatic nucleus (SCN) (see page 246) and affected by environmental cues, known as *zeitgebers*, that include light and darkness, these rhythms regulate many physiological processes, including sleep and wake cycles.[5] Other cues, like temperature and hormones, also help set these clocks at the cellular level.[6]

Over the past 20 years, we've gained significant insights into these clocks. They are so important that in 2017, Jeffrey C. Hall, Michael Rosbach and Michael W. Young were awarded a Nobel Prize for discovering the molecular mechanisms controlling circadian rhythms.[7]

These clocks regulate sleep, mood, energy levels, digestion and cognitive function. However, modern living often disrupts these rhythms, negatively impacting health. Dysregulation can lead to mood swings, cognitive impairments, hormonal imbalances, metabolic issues, increased disease risks and reduced immunity. Indoor lifestyles and artificial lighting have given us a 24/7 world – but at what cost?

Pause and reflect

Pause for a moment and reflect on your relationship with time. How much of your life is dictated by the clock rather than your internal rhythms? When free from external demands, do you naturally adopt healthier habits or struggle with self-regulation?

Hold on to these thoughts as we explore the profound impact of time and routine on our lives.

Chronotype: Are you a morning or night person?

Your chronotype refers to your body's natural preference for being a morning person (lark) or a night person (owl). Multiple genes, including the PER3 gene, help determine these preferences. Genetic tests can provide insights based on genetic markers associated with sleep patterns. However, these tests suggest tendencies rather than definitive answers. Beyond genetics, factors like environment, lifestyle, time zone and personal habits influence your sleep patterns.

How the population splits into chronotypes:

While most people fall into one of three broad categories – there is a spectrum within each group, with individuals leaning more or less strongly towards their type.

- Morning types (larks): About 10–20 per cent of people are morning types.
- Intermediate types: 60–70 per cent fall somewhere in between.
- Evening types (owls): 20–30 per cent are evening types.[8]
- There are degrees of variation within each chronotype. For example, an extreme morning type might naturally wake at 4 a.m., regardless of external obligations, while an extreme evening type may not fall asleep until around 3 a.m. and wake at midday, struggling to align with conventional schedules. Intermediate types may lean slightly towards morning or evening preferences but tend to remain more adaptable overall.

For some, especially those with extreme chronotypes, the traditional 9-to-5 schedule becomes a persistent challenge, often leading to chronic sleep deprivation and its associated health and performance consequences. Night owls, in particular, face disadvantages as their natural rhythms frequently conflict with societal expectations, leaving them at odds with both work and social commitments.[9]

Historically, diverse sleep patterns within a community may have ensured someone was always awake to keep watch. Today, recognising and respecting these natural differences can improve personal and social wellbeing, allowing individuals to tailor their schedules to better fit their own rhythms.

Our natural sleep patterns aren't set in stone, but it's tough for a night owl to become an early bird. People's sleep preferences can vary by up to ten hours between those who wake up very early ('larks') and those who stay up late ('owls'). During the teenage years, our internal clock shifts later, peaking around age 19.5 for women and 21 for men and often persisting into their mid-twenties. This biological delay, known as delayed sleep phase syndrome (DSPS), makes it nearly impossible for many teens to fall asleep early enough to wake up refreshed for early school or work schedules. Forcing them into these patterns is not just frustrating – it's damaging. Studies show this shift is real, and it's harder for teens to fall asleep early because their bodies produce melatonin, the sleep hormone, later at night.

By the time we reach our 50s and 60s, our sleep patterns naturally shift earlier again. Still, for those who remain night owls or are affected by neurodiversity – such as individuals with ADHD or autism – these challenges don't go away. Neurodivergent people are often more likely to experience delayed sleep–wake cycles, meaning they face additional hurdles navigating a world designed for early risers.

A small UK study showed how by implementing the following protocols for night owls, cognitive (reaction time) and physical (grip strength) performance measures improved, with peak performance shifting from evening to afternoon. Those night owls also ate breakfast more frequently and reported better mental wellbeing, with reduced stress and depression.[10] I recommend making the time shifts incrementally so that you don't run into the problem of trying to go to sleep when you are not sleepy or waking up and triggering sleep inertia.

How to be less of a night owl

- Gradually start waking up earlier, aiming to eventually wake up two to three hours before your usual time, and spend as much time as possible in natural sunlight during the morning.

- Similarly, begin adjusting your bedtime earlier in small increments, working towards going to bed two to three hours before your current bedtime. To help with this, reduce light exposure in the evening.
- Keep your sleep and wake times consistent every day, including weekends, to support this shift.
- Eat breakfast soon after waking, establish a consistent lunchtime and try to finish dinner by 7 p.m. to reinforce your new schedule.

When things like early school start times go against our natural sleep rhythms, it can cause sleep deprivation. This lack of sleep can lead to poor grades, mental health problems and a higher risk of accidents.[11] It's remarkable that more isn't made of this when you consider the rising tide of anxiety and depression in our teens, with 38 per cent of youth experiencing anxiety and 3.1 per cent experiencing depression at least once by age 14.[12] Some schools have experimented with later start times to address this issue, but more research is needed.[13] Wholesale change is complex, and it doesn't work for all teenagers. So, while technology use plays a role in sleep disruption, this biological mismatch is the biggest issue.

Understanding your chronotype

Understanding your chronotype – whether you're a morning person, a night owl or somewhere in between – can help you optimise your daily routine and improve your sleep. A chronotype questionnaire is a simple tool that can help you identify your natural sleep–wake preferences.

There are many questionnaires available online, but if you'd like to look into specific ones, the below are the most frequently used:

Munich Chronotype Questionnaire (MCTQ):[14] This question-naire is widely used in sleep research to assess chronotypes based on your preferred sleep times on workdays and free days.

Morningness-Eveningness Questionnaire (MEQ):[15] The MEQ is another common tool that evaluates whether you're more of a morning or evening person based on your daily routines.

Consistency – the key piece in the sleep jigsaw

It's not just about how much sleep you get – it's about keeping a consistent sleep schedule that aligns with your chronotype. A study using data from the UK Biobank explored this by tracking the sleep patterns of over 60,000 people in their 50s, 60s and 70s over at least five days. Participants wore actigraphy devices on their wrists to monitor movement and objectively measure sleep and wake times. They also kept sleep diaries and completed questionnaires to give researchers a fuller picture of their habits.

Researchers developed a Sleep Regularity Index (SRI) to measure consistency, where a higher score indicated more stable sleep patterns. The results were striking: people with the most regular sleep schedules – those who went to bed and woke up at the same time every day – were over 30 per cent less likely to die during the nearly eight-year follow-up period than those with the most irregular patterns.[16] The takeaway? Consistency isn't just a tiny detail – it can make a significant difference.

The myth of the 5 a.m. mindset

I recall headlines about former British Prime Minister Rishi Sunak's morning routine and empathised with his team, who had to arrive at No. 10 'hours early'[17] to get on top of their work in line with his early bird tendencies.

As we learn more about diverse sleep patterns, it becomes clear for many people that the early-rising practice is flawed. While a consistent morning wake-up time can anchor your sleep schedule, it doesn't have to be at the crack of dawn. For night owls, rising early is not just challenging;

it's a profound misalignment with their natural rhythms and can lead to poor health. Instead, consider how structuring your routine based on how you feel might improve your life.

Not everyone has the luxury of choosing when to wake up. Many are constrained by demanding jobs, financial pressures or caregiving responsibilities. For them, the advice to wake up at 5 a.m. is impractical and dismissive of their realities. While Rishi Sunak was the prime minister, he is also a father. Ignoring his personal financial situation, if one partner follows this early schedule, where does that leave the other? This highlights a broader issue of privilege, where early rising becomes another unattainable standard, increasing stress among those who can't comply.

Given the rise in sleep-related disorders, embracing our natural rhythms could significantly improve health and wellbeing. It's time for a more nuanced understanding of productivity – one that values authentic living, embraces human diversity and acknowledges the realities of those without the privilege of choice.

Spring forward, fall back

Think about how jet lag makes you feel when you travel across time zones – tired and out of sync because your internal clock is misaligned with the new local time. This disruption is a typical example of circadian dysregulation. Staying up late or waking up early against your natural sleep pattern can cause a similar feeling. A common instance of circadian dysregulation is daylight saving time, affecting about a quarter of people worldwide. In spring, clocks 'spring forward', causing you to lose an hour. In autumn, clocks 'fall back', giving you an extra hour in bed.

Daylight saving time was first proposed by British builder William Willett (1856–1915), who was passionate about using daylight more efficiently. In his 1907 pamphlet, *The Waste of Daylight*,[18] Willett suggested advancing clocks by 80 minutes in spring and reversing them in autumn. Despite introducing multiple bills to Parliament, his efforts faced opposition from farmers and those concerned about disruptions. Willett passed away in 1915, never seeing his idea adopted.

World War I changed that. Germany introduced DST in 1916 to conserve coal, prompting the UK to follow with the Summer Time Act 1916, adopting a one-hour clock change. Today, DST remains debated, with advocates citing energy savings and safety benefits, while critics, especially in northern regions, highlight the challenges of darker mornings.

An interesting connection? Willett's great-great-grandson is Coldplay's Chris Martin, and some speculate the opening lyrics of 'Clocks' – 'the lights go out and I can't be saved' – may reference DST.[19]

The subtle stress caused by DST may not be immediately apparent, but it does affect us.[20] Waking up an hour earlier than usual increases the risk of health issues like heart problems, weakened immune systems, injuries and mental health disorders. Night owls are particularly affected, taking longer to adapt when clocks move forward in spring, increasing their cardiovascular risks and stress levels.

The days following the spring forward have been linked to severe consequences, including a rise in heart attacks, strokes, immune system problems and accidents. The arguments whether to keep DST have been going backwards and forwards for over 100 years. Given these findings, there is growing consensus that DST should be abandoned. In the UK, the Royal Society for the Prevention of Accidents has called for this change, arguing that DST increases the risk of road accidents, with studies showing a significant increase in fatal traffic accidents (up to 30 per cent on the first day).[21] Ideally, social schedules would align with our internal rhythms and the sun's natural cycle. DST disrupts this harmony, nudging our biological rhythms off course.

How to handle this time shift

How do you navigate this shift until a more permanent solution is found? It's wise to step more cautiously during the DST transition periods.

- When we lose an hour in the spring, be extra vigilant on the roads.
- Consider going to bed 10 to 15 minutes earlier each night leading up to the change to ease the transition.
- Getting some morning sunlight can help adjust your internal clock to the new time, making it a bit easier to wake up.

Weekend time hops

When weekends feel like crossing multiple time zones, it's not just your imagination. Your body experiences something akin to social jet lag if you drastically change your sleep schedule from weekday to weekend. While staying up late on Friday and Saturday nights is tempting, try not to stray too far from your regular sleep routine. If you stay up late, don't worry on Sunday night; adjusting will take a couple of days.

If you usually get seven or eight hours of sleep per night but drop to around five hours on the weekends, you accumulate a sleep debt of five hours by Monday. This sleep debt makes it harder to wake up early during the workweek, making your routine more challenging.

The key is establishing a routine and sticking to it. Even if weekends offer more flexibility, try not to shift too much from your regular sleep schedule. It's fine to stay up a little later for fun, but still ensure you get enough rest. This approach helps minimise the effects of social jet lag and makes it easier to transition back into your weekday rhythm.

For some people, especially those with circadian rhythm disorders, adjusting to society's 9-to-5 schedule can be even more difficult. There is more information on when and how sleep timing can be a biological problem in Chapter Seven.

How to pay off a sleep debt

You will not pay it down in one go, e.g. going to bed early on Sunday night to recoup the cost. Instead, short naps of 20–30 minutes on Saturday and Sunday afternoons could mitigate some of the sleep loss without disrupting your night-time sleep, but avoid long naps, especially late in the day. You could also steadily pay the debt down by increasing your sleep time by 15 to 30 minutes.

Zeitgebers: the keys to synchronising your rhythms

To set yourself up for a good night's sleep, the secret lies in the signals you send your body throughout the day. *Zeitgebers*, a German term meaning 'time givers' or 'synchronisers', are environmental cues – such as light exposure, meal timing and physical activity – that help regulate your body's internal clock. These cues send signals to your brain and major organs, keeping your circadian rhythms in sync with the outside world.

Light is the most powerful *zeitgeber* we have, because it directly influences the release of melatonin, the hormone that helps regulate sleep. When you get bright, natural light in the morning, it sends a clear signal to your brain that it's time to be awake and alert. Without that signal, especially in winter or on overcast days, your body can feel sluggish and misaligned, as if you're operating in a different time zone.

Without the clear signal of light to jumpstart your day, it can feel like you're dragging yourself out of bed into an endless grey fog. Using a daylight alarm clock or a light therapy box becomes essential, simulating the sunlight you're missing. By exposing yourself to bright light early in the day, you're essentially 'setting' your internal clock, making it easier to feel awake in the morning and tired in the evening.

Adding consistent cues throughout your morning routine can reinforce these signals. Eating breakfast within an hour of waking up, for example, serves as a secondary *zeitgeber* that tells your body the day has started. When you eat at regular times each day, your digestive system syncs up with your body's other rhythms, helping you feel more energised and focused.

Other aspects of daily life, like the timing of bathroom breaks, can also serve as subtle but effective *zeitgebers*. Going to the bathroom at predictable times – first thing in the morning, after meals and before bed – adds an extra layer of regularity to your day. These small, routine actions might seem trivial, but they contribute to the stability your body craves, reinforcing the timing of your internal clock.

While it's less about something that you do at the same time every day, it is something to be aware of, especially if you take exercise close to bedtime. As evening approaches, your body's core temperature naturally begins to drop, signalling that it's time to wind down. This cooling process is a critical part of preparing for sleep. You can support it by lowering the room temperature in the evening or taking a warm bath about an hour before bed. The warm water increases blood flow to your skin, which helps dissipate heat more quickly when you step out, leading to a faster drop in core temperature. This temperature shift can make you feel sleepy and helps you fall asleep more easily.

By doing the same things at the same time every day – like getting bright light in the morning, eating meals on a schedule and being aware of temperature at night – you reduce mental effort and support your circadian rhythm. These small, consistent actions work together to help you fall asleep more easily, wake up refreshed and boost your energy throughout the day. Over time, consistency turns these intentional habits into effortless routines.

Everything everywhere, all at once

Many of us are fortunate to live in a world where food is always within reach, no matter where we are. This constant availability has led many of us to eat throughout the day, disrupting our body's natural rhythms. Professor Satchidananda Panda explores this issue in his book, *The Circadian Code*. He explains how our modern eating habits can cause metabolic problems like obesity, diabetes and heart disease.

Professor Panda suggests a solution called time-restricted eating (TRE). This involves consuming all your daily calories within an 8–12-hour window.[22] Doing this can align your eating patterns with your body's natural rhythms, improving overall health. When you eat, sensors in your gut detect changes such as blood sugar levels and the release of hormones like insulin and ghrelin. These sensors send signals to your brain, helping to regulate your body's biological clock.

Additionally, aligning mealtimes with your biological clock may improve sleep quality.[23] However, it's important to note that TRE might not suit everyone, so finding an eating pattern that works for you is best.[24]

Get social

In our increasingly isolated world, staying connected to others is more important than ever. Spending time with people you trust – friends, family, those who see you and understand you – does more than lift your spirits. It engages the parts of your brain tied to social behaviour and emotions, like the prefrontal cortex and limbic system. These interactions help synchronise your internal rhythms, grounding you in a sense of belonging and emotional wellbeing.

But as artificial intelligence steps into the realm of companionship, offering digital 'friends' and virtual interactions, it raises some big questions. How will these AI-generated relationships affect us – not just in terms of social withdrawal, but in the deeper ways they might change our experience of connection? Early research suggests that while AI companions can ease loneliness or reduce stress, as yet, they can't offer the genuine empathy or the subtle comfort that human interactions provide.

There's something irreplaceable about being physically present with others. When you're face-to-face with someone, you experience the full richness of connection: you can see the shifts in their body language, hear the nuances in their voice and feel the warmth of a touch. These sensory experiences are powerful – they're what create real, lasting bonds. Digital interactions, no matter how advanced, can currently only imitate this depth, but I am curious to see where technology takes us. Human connection fulfils a need that goes beyond words, beyond algorithms; it speaks to a primal part of you that craves closeness, understanding and presence.

Jean, 32, has become increasingly reclusive and estranged from her social group, leading to anxiety and disrupted sleep. Her argument with a best friend, primarily over text, exacerbates her insomnia, causing her to compulsively check her phone at night. 'I have had a huge argument with my best friend,' she explains. 'It started over text and just spiralled out of control. We haven't seen each other in person for months; we only talk via text, but it's getting worse. I can't sleep and I'm worried I'm going to lose her.'

This story highlights a modern struggle where the convenience of digital communication leads to isolation and begins to undermine our wellbeing. The situation underscores how time – both the amount of time spent in certain activities and the time of day – plays a role in our mental and emotional health. The time Jean spends anxiously waiting for a response, especially late at night, not only disrupts her sleep but also her circadian rhythm. Her GP prescribed temporary sleeping pills, but as Jean herself realised, these were not addressing the root of the problem.

'I've tried to explain, but every time I text, it make it worse,' Jean says. 'She has stopped replying, and I find myself compulsively texting, watching the three dots appear as if she's going to reply, but nothing comes. It's like time stands still.'

I asked Jean if she had considered trying to resolve this face-to-face. She nods slowly. 'If only we could, but she says she's too busy. The more we text, the more misunderstood I feel, and it's making me more anxious and sleepless. I wake up repeatedly, checking my phone to see if she has replied.'

This is the crux of Jean's dilemma: the amount of time spent in fruitless digital exchanges not only wastes precious hours that could be spent resting but also extends the emotional turmoil into the night. The absence of physical presence in these interactions means that critical non-verbal cues – those subtle signals of empathy, understanding and connection – are lost, leading to more misunderstandings and prolonged conflict.

While digital interactions can help maintain connections when in-person meetings aren't possible, they can't fully replace the depth needed for real emotional connection. While many people thrive on solitude, spending up to 75 per cent of their time alone without feeling isolated,[25] this equilibrium is closely tied to the quality of their relationships and support networks. Jean's situation highlights how a lack of meaningful face-to-face interaction can disrupt this dynamic, increasing stress and affecting sleep.

Jean's experience highlights the importance of not only managing the *amount* of time spent on communication but also being deliberate about *when* in the day we engage. By reserving her late-night hours for rest and winding down rather than for online conflict, Jean could reclaim those precious minutes before bed and allow her mind to reset. The stress from unresolved conflicts and the absence of face-to-face interactions have taken a toll on her emotional and social rest, which in turn affects her sleep. Addressing her social needs and prioritising direct, meaningful interaction – spending time in person rather than online – could help alleviate her anxiety and improve her sleep quality.

Ultimately, time is more than a measure of the clock; it's a resource that, when spent wisely, can either restore or deplete our mental and emotional reserves. By reclaiming her evening hours for rest rather than digital distractions, Jean could find not only better sleep but also greater emotional equanimity.

Movement matters

We've discussed using exercise as an outlet for anger, but it can also be a powerful antidote to loneliness and a boon for sleep, especially when it's something you actually enjoy. Moving your body should feel good, not like another chore on the list. When you find movement that's fun – whether it's dancing, hiking or a game of tennis – you're far more likely to keep it up, reaping both physical and mental benefits along the way.

Social exercise – joining a gym, a sports team or a community class – can add a sense of camaraderie and belonging. These connections foster inclusion, ease loneliness and boost mood through shared experience. Physical activity also releases endorphins – natural mood lifters that make us feel more alive, connected and resilient.

Beyond the social and emotional perks, regularly timed exercise is a key *zeitgeber* that helps regulate your body clock. And it doesn't need to be intense to be effective; it just needs to be something you look forward to. When movement feels enjoyable, you'll find yourself coming back to it again and again. Even lighter activities like walking, stretching or gardening can help reduce stress, boost energy and prepare your body for restful sleep.

Regular movement also benefits your joints by boosting the production of synovial fluid, which keeps them lubricated and healthy. This is especially important as we age, since joint stiffness and aches can easily disrupt sleep. The simple truth is: keep moving to keep your joints comfortable and reduce the risk of discomfort that can disturb your night.

Recent research shows that combining aerobic exercise with resistance training improves sleep quality, particularly in older adults. In one study, participants followed a 12-week programme, engaging in moderate-intensity exercise twice a week in the evening, and gradually increasing their daily steps. By the end, they were moving more, sleeping better,[26] and feeling an overall lift in mood and wellbeing.

Feeling sluggish? Take a walk – and make it fun

When that afternoon slump hits, skip the coffee and step outside for a quick walk. Make it something you enjoy – take a scenic route, listen to music you love or bring a friend along.

Studies show that regular walks, especially in green spaces, reduce symptoms of depression and anxiety, helping you wind down more easily at night. Physically, walking strengthens your heart, supports weight management and can even protect against sleep disturbances like sleep apnea. Aiming for 10,000 steps a day – a goal popularised in Japan in the 1960s[27] – is more than just a fitness trend; it's a way to keep your body and mind in sync.

Walking outside also exposes you to natural light, a key factor in regulating your sleep–wake cycle. Most of us spend up to 90 per cent of our time indoors, missing out on this essential cue that aligns our circadian rhythm. Morning walks are especially effective, setting you up for better energy during the day and deeper sleep at night.

Adding more movement doesn't have to be a grind. NEAT (non-exercise activity thermogenesis) refers to the energy expended through activities other than deliberate exercise, such as daily tasks, movements and spontaneous physical activities. Even fidgeting contributes – tapping your foot, drumming your fingers or shifting in your seat fall into this category because they involve low-intensity movement that contributes to overall energy expenditure.

Ask yourself: where can you bring more movement – and more fun – into your routine? Turn a meeting into a walk-and-talk. Crank up your favourite song while you tidy up the house. If you work from home, dance while waiting for the kettle to boil. It's not about carving out hours for exercise but finding little pockets of fun and movement throughout your day.

The beauty of this habit is that it's a positive cycle: when you move, you sleep better; when you sleep well, you have more energy to move. And remember, movement can be gentle and adaptable to your needs – it's about keeping your body in motion, whatever that looks like for you.

The more seamlessly you weave movement into your life, the more likely you are to stick with it. So, start small, keep it fun and notice how much better you feel, especially when it's time to rest.

Light up your days

Your body is a master timekeeper, attuned to the rhythms of the earth without the need for a watch. The secret lies in light – the primary *zeitgeber* that synchronises our biological clocks, influencing everything from sleep to mood to mental clarity. But in today's world, we've become indoor creatures, waking before dawn, commuting in darkness and spending our days under artificial lighting. This modern lifestyle disrupts our natural rhythms, leading to difficulty falling asleep, waking up, and even contributing to increased stress, anxiety and depression.

Over 80 per cent of the body's metabolic processes follow a daily pattern – active during the day, less active at night. Natural light helps keep these processes running smoothly. Unlike indoor lighting, which is often too dim to have a significant impact, sunlight provides the necessary intensity to stimulate melanopsin, a pigment in our eyes that helps regulate our internal clocks.

Imagine stepping outside on a sunny day, where sunlight can range from 10,000 to 100,000 lux, compared with the mere 100 to 500 lux of typical indoor lighting. How does it make you feel? Here in the UK where much of our winters are an unremitting shade of grey, sunlight is a welcome lift to the general mood.

This difference is vital, especially as we age. By age 45, your eyes receive only half the light they did in your youth, making natural light exposure even more critical for regulating your internal clock.

Personally, as a night owl, I struggle with sleep inertia in the mornings, waking up groggy and unfocused. It wasn't until I became a dog owner and started taking morning walks that I noticed a change. The morning light not only woke me up but also lifted my mood and set a positive tone for the day. It was as if the light itself was coaching me through the day, gently pushing me to stay in sync with the world around me.

A loss of light

A growing trend among young people shows a worrying connection between reduced exposure to natural light and rising mental health issues. A 2024 study from the Resolution Foundation revealed that

34 per cent of young people aged 18 to 24 reported symptoms of mental disorders like depression and anxiety in 2021/22, up from 24 per cent in 2000.[28] Consequently, over half a million individuals in this age group were prescribed antidepressants during the same period. There is a significant connection between reduced exposure to natural light and the increasing rates of mental health issues. Shockingly, this same group reported spending only 30 minutes outside daily.

This issue isn't isolated to young people. An American survey found that 58.8 per cent of people spend one hour or less per day outdoors, with 37.4 per cent getting 30 minutes or less, and 18.3 per cent spending under 15 minutes outside daily. Women are particularly affected, with 45.4 per cent of women versus 29.1 per cent of men spending 30 minutes or less outdoors. Women are also 64 per cent more likely to spend only 15 minutes or less outside.[29]

How to use light to your benefit:

- Take short breaks outside throughout the day. Aim for at least 30 minutes of outdoor time each day.
- Position your workspace near a window or take walking meetings to soak up daylight.
- Integrate outdoor hobbies like walking, jogging, or gardening into your routine.
- Set up a balcony or garden space to enjoy the sun at home. Even sitting on your doorstep or throwing open the windows can help.
- In winter, go outside during midday when the sun is highest. In summer, take advantage of the early morning or late afternoon sun.
- Seek out parks or community spaces where you feel comfortable spending time.
- Using blackout curtains or an eye mask to block external lights and reducing screen time before bed can also help. Morning light exposure is needed for a natural waking cycle.

- Light-based alarm clocks can provide a more gentle and natural way to wake up, reducing sleep inertia and promoting a healthier start to the day.

The impact of geography on circadian rhythms

How your body responds to light also depends on where you live. Near the equator, you experience a consistent cycle of day and night throughout the year. The sun rises and sets at almost the same time each day, providing a steady, predictable rhythm that your body can easily adapt to.

Further from the equator, however, the story changes. Days stretch long in the summer and shrink dramatically in winter, throwing off the natural cues your body relies on. Dark mornings in winter and lingering summer sunsets can disrupt your natural rhythm, making it difficult to maintain a regular sleep pattern and leading to a general sense of unease.

The advent of electricity has had a radical impact on environmental light levels, with many who live in urban settings never experiencing true darkness, let alone seeing the stars at night. Yet we need darkness for our sleep. Light and dark both have powerful impacts on our health.

Different cultures have developed unique practices to maintain wellbeing in low-light conditions. For example, in Scandinavia, the concept of *'friluftsliv'* (open-air living) is embraced even in the harshest winters. Meanwhile, in India, sunrise yoga is a practice that aligns the body with the rhythm of the day.

So, what can you do? I would love that we follow nature and hibernate/slow down in the winter months, but life won't allow us that luxury. Start your day with light, let it guide you, energise you and keep your rhythms synchronised. If you can't access natural light, use a lightbox (see below).

In the evening, as the light fades – or even if it doesn't – keep lights low and take a mindful approach to devices. Aim for darkness in your sleep space – it is the most important signal for your body to know it's nighttime, triggering sleep-promoting mechanisms. Light exposure at night can confuse this system, disrupting your sleep and overall energy balance.

In a world that often feels too fast and too artificial, let the simple act of stepping into the light reconnect you with your natural rhythm – one that is as old as time itself.

Light boxes

We often use 10,000-lux lightboxes to treat circadian rhythm disorders and seasonal affective disorder (SAD). Standard protocols involve daily exposure to bright light for 30 to 60 minutes, with consistency being key for effectiveness.[30] Bright light therapy (BLT) was first introduced in 1984 as a treatment for SAD and is particularly effective for individuals who struggle to get enough natural light.[31] However, responses to light therapy can vary, and when addressing circadian rhythm disorders, it's essential to determine whether the goal is to shift the body clock forward or backward. A professional consultation is recommended to create a personalised treatment plan.

Chronotype-specific recommendations:

Early risers – morning larks: If you naturally wake up and go to bed early, you benefit from getting plenty of morning sunlight. This helps you stay in sync with your sleep routine.[32]

Late risers – night owls: If you tend to stay up late and sleep in, it helps to gradually get more morning light and reduce evening light. This can make it easier to align your sleep schedule with the rest of the world.[33]

In-between types – intermediate chronotypes: Most people fall somewhere between early risers and late risers. To keep your sleep on track, try to get some sunlight in the morning and throughout the day.[34]

Understanding the timing and effects of light exposure can help manage your sleep–wake cycle more effectively. Bright light at night can delay your bedtime and wake-up time, making it harder to fall asleep and wake up at usual times. Conversely, bright light in the morning can help you wake up earlier and feel more refreshed. Shift workers face unique challenges in maintaining a healthy light–dark cycle. Irregular work hours can disrupt their natural sleep–wake cycle, leading to sleep disorders, fatigue and impaired cognitive function. Strategic light exposure, such as bright light during night shifts to stay alert and darkness during the day to aid sleep, can benefit shift workers.

Light anxiety

Fear of the dark, known formally as achluophobia, and its more intense counterpart, nyctophobia, can be a big problem at any age. Historically, darkness signified danger, providing cover for predators and other threats. This primal fear of the unknown and unseen has served as a survival mechanism, potentially passed down through generations.

The inability to see in the dark naturally triggers anxiety, a deeply ingrained response as the brain is wired to protect us from potential harm. Light plays a vital role in calming the amygdala, the brain's fear centre, and strengthening its connection with the prefrontal cortex, which helps manage emotions. This neurological reaction may explain our modern preference for well-lit environments and frequent use of electronic devices. The sense of safety and control that light provides is indeed powerful.

Our fear of the dark is not solely evolutionary; psychological factors also play a significant role. Watching frightening or violent media before bed can amplify irrational fears that darkness exacerbates. Traumatic childhood experiences can linger into adulthood as nyctophobia. Sometimes, this fear arises without any apparent trigger and may require professional intervention, especially if nightmares or night terrors become a problem.

Stressful or traumatic events, genetics, and exposure to anxious or overprotective caregivers in childhood can increase the likelihood of fearing the dark. While many find solace in some light at night, others prefer complete darkness to sleep. This preference for total darkness is common and can significantly enhance sleep quality for those who find even minimal light disruptive. However, there's a difference between a simple preference for darkness and an intense aversion to light, which can be linked to conditions like scotophobia or lygophobia – a fear of light.

For some individuals, this intense need for darkness goes beyond preference.[35] These individuals may travel with gaffer tape and blackout fabric to cover every stray light source in hotel rooms, ensuring that no light disrupts their sleep environment. This heightened sensitivity to light can be deeply intertwined with conditions like insomnia or anxiety disorders. For them, even the tiniest glimmer can trigger a sense of alertness and discomfort, making relaxation and sleep seem nearly impossible. This reaction often reflects a deeper need for control and predictability in their environment, where total darkness provides a sanctuary that allows them to finally let their guard down and rest.

So, while many people simply enjoy sleeping in darkness for comfort, those with an intense sensitivity to light might require total darkness to manage their anxiety and ensure a restful night's sleep. Understanding this distinction is key to addressing individual sleep needs and creating an environment conducive to rest, whether that means total darkness or simply minimising light to a comfortable level.

The cortisol/melatonin seesaw

Many people say to me they have tried to use melatonin as a sleeping pill but it didn't work – this is because that isn't what it is. Melatonin is a sleep hormone that signals to your body that it's time to start winding down for the night. It's a subtle nudge, not a knockout punch.

It really highlights the interlinked nature of your biology. Melatonin is closely linked to cortisol which peaks in the morning. Around 12–14 hours after that cortisol peak, the body starts producing melatonin, prepping you for sleep. These two hormones are like a seesaw: when cortisol is high in the morning, melatonin is low, keeping you awake. As cortisol drops in the evening, melatonin rises, setting the stage for sleep.

This is why having a consistent wake-up time matters so much. When you get up at the same time every day, you're anchoring your cortisol peak, which in turn helps to stabilise your melatonin production in the evening. If your wake time is all over the place, your whole sleep–wake cycle can get thrown off, making it harder to fall asleep when you want to.

A common mistake people make is taking a melatonin supplement at odd times, like in the middle of the night – around 3 a.m., for example. By this point, your body's natural melatonin cycle is already tapering off as it prepares for morning wakefulness. Taking melatonin at that hour might temporarily make you feel drowsy, but it can also confuse your body's natural rhythm, making it harder to sleep consistently over time. Instead of addressing the root cause of your early wake-ups, it may actually disrupt your sleep cycle further.

In the UK, you need a prescription for melatonin supplements. If you're buying melatonin from abroad, be careful – some products might have way more melatonin in them than they claim, sometimes up to five times more.[36] It's always safer to go with products that have been verified by trusted sources.[37]

Generally speaking, melatonin is safe – it's not addictive and doesn't cause serious side effects for most people. But you need to take it in the correct way for the right reasons. It's not recommended for teenagers going through puberty or for people taking certain medications. So, as always, it's a good idea to talk to your doctor before you start taking melatonin or any other sleep aid.

Scrambled rhythms

Jet lag and shift work both disrupt your circadian rhythm, leaving you feeling foggy and out of sync because your internal clock hasn't adjusted to the new schedule. Melatonin can be used strategically to help reset this rhythm in situations like these.

The key to using it effectively for jet lag lies in timing. When you cross time zones, your body needs help resetting its internal clock, and melatonin can be that gentle nudge. But it's not about taking it as soon as you feel tired – it's about using it strategically. For example, if you're travelling eastward – from New York to Paris – you might take melatonin in the early evening at your destination to help your body adjust to the new time zone.

On the flip side, westward travel is generally easier on your body. Our circadian rhythms naturally lean towards slightly longer days, so adjusting to a longer wakefulness period comes more naturally. Imagine flying from Los Angeles to Tokyo: your body prefers to stay awake longer rather than go to bed earlier. Taking melatonin a few hours before your desired bedtime at your destination can help you transition smoothly.

To make this adjustment even easier, apps like Timeshifter offer personalised jet lag plans based on your travel itinerary and sleep patterns. These tools give practical tips on when to expose yourself to light, when to avoid it, and when to take melatonin, all of which can make your transition to a new time zone less jarring.

Now, let's address the dreaded red-eye flight – a notorious challenge for your circadian rhythm. Imagine flying from the East Coast of the US to London, arriving early in the morning. Your body thinks it's the middle of the night, but the sun is rising at your destination. Like so many of us trying to squeeze every hour out of our schedule, you might go straight to work after landing. This is where things get tricky – the body's natural rhythms are completely misaligned, and you might be running on little to no sleep. For many, this leads to reduced alertness, poor judgement and reduced problem-solving abilities. These effects aren't just inconvenient, they can be dangerous, especially in high-pressure environments where decisions have significant consequences.

This practice of pushing through without rest also highlights a broader cultural issue. So often work and productivity take priority over personal health and wellbeing. But expecting someone to transition seamlessly from a long flight directly into a full day of work without recovery time is a recipe for mistakes, lower productivity and even accidents. It ignores your body's basic needs.

Interestingly, the misalignment you experience on a red-eye flight is similar to what night owls – especially teenagers – face daily. We have explored how their body clocks change during puberty and into early adulthood. This delayed rhythm means they're often functioning in a state of chronic misalignment, which can lead to the same cognitive impairments and health risks that we associate with jet lag.

Night owls might think they have an edge when it comes to red-eye flights because they're naturally inclined to stay up later. But don't be fooled – night owls aren't immune to jet lag or adjusting to a new time zone. They'll still face the same difficulties syncing their body clock to local time, even if the initial impact isn't as severe.

To keep your mind sharp and stay healthy, can you rest after long flights instead of diving straight into work? Your body needs time to catch up; respecting this process will help you recover more quickly and perform better in the long run.

The shift-work struggle

With our 24/7 world, more people are working night shifts than ever before – around 8.7 million in the UK alone,[38] including blue light workers, construction crews and warehouse staff. And even if you don't consider yourself a shift worker, you might still be affected by the ripple effects of shift work in ways you haven't realised. Maybe it's your partner, a friend or a neighbour whose unusual hours impact your life. Have you ever thought blasting music during your 10 a.m. workout might disturb someone trying to sleep after a long night shift? We all know people who work shifts – doctors, nurses, factory workers, emergency responders – or maybe you manage a team with people who directly or indirectly work shifts. But do we truly understand their experience? Imagine trying to stay awake all night when your body is screaming for rest, only to see the sunrise when you're supposed to wind down. It's not just about being tired; it's about living in constant biological chaos.

I recall meeting a DJ who relished his unconventional schedule. A night owl by nature, he embraced the high-energy hours of his work, enjoying a lifestyle that allowed him to sleep from 6 a.m. to 3 p.m. His partner got home at 6 p.m., and they enjoyed their evenings together before he headed off to work at 10 p.m. They made it work because their timing was consistent – they both knew where they stood. That consistency made a difference, both psychologically and biologically. But in the dance between professional demands and biological needs, many shift workers – especially those whose shift timings often change – feel out of step, leading to a profound sense of disconnection from their bodies and the world around them. This dance has inspired numerous attempts to create better systems, yet no solution has fully addressed the circadian disruptions it causes.

The broader impact of disrupted rhythms

Shift workers often sleep less than seven hours a day, grappling with issues like insomnia, excessive sleepiness (hypersomnia), microsleeps – brief, unintentional lapses into sleep – alongside depression, fatigue and trouble concentrating. These aren't just inconveniences; they're signs that your body's natural rhythm is being disrupted.

The consequences of working against your circadian rhythm can be profound. While it might feel like you're adapting to night shifts after a few weeks, this 'adjustment' is deceptive. Our bodies never fully adapt to being active at night. The human body operates on a natural sleep–wake cycle that aligns closely with the day–night pattern, signalling when to be alert and when to wind down. Even if you feel like you've adjusted, the health risks associated with misaligned sleep schedules don't simply disappear.

After a night shift, exposure to light – whether from daylight on your way home or artificial lighting indoors – sends a powerful signal to your brain that it's time to stay awake, interfering with melatonin production. Even if you're physically exhausted, elevated adrenaline and cortisol from a demanding shift can leave you feeling 'wired', making it difficult to relax and drift off to sleep.

To counteract these effects, shift workers often need to adopt specific strategies to help their bodies wind down after work, like using black-out curtains, avoiding caffeine, or practising relaxation techniques. But sometimes, these strategies aren't enough. When the ongoing struggle to manage your work hours creates a persistent cycle of sleep deprivation and fatigue, it could signal a deeper issue – a medical condition that deserves attention. Shift work sleep disorder (SWSD) is a circadian rhythm sleep disorder that affects people who work nonstandard hours. If you struggle to stay awake during your shifts or cannot sleep even when you're exhausted, SWSD might be at the root of the problem. For more information, see page 247. Equally, while shift work plays a significant role in sleep health, it's not always the only cause of sleep problems. If you are a shift worker, identifying whether you have a sleep disorder and treating it is not just about shift working.

Beware the vending machine

One particularly alarming finding is how shift work affects glucose metabolism by disrupting the body's circadian rhythms. The circadian misalignment impairs glucose tolerance, which can significantly raise the risk of type 2 diabetes.[39]

Disrupted sleep patterns also mess with your hormones, contributing to weight gain and obesity. On page 101, we have seen how, when you don't get enough sleep, levels of the hormone ghrelin, which makes you feel hungry, go up, while leptin, the hormone that signals fullness, goes down. This imbalance often leads to overeating, particularly cravings for high-calorie, carb-heavy foods – which, unfortunately, are usually what's available in vending machines during those late-night shifts.

And here's where things can get even trickier. Obesity itself is a major risk factor for obstructive sleep apnea (OSA), a condition that causes your airway to become blocked during sleep, leading to frequent interruptions in breathing. When already dealing with the challenges of irregular sleep, the onset of sleep apnea creates a bigger problem.

The cycle goes like this: weight gain due to disrupted metabolic processes increases the likelihood of developing sleep apnea. Sleep apnea further fragments your sleep, making you more tired during the day. This fatigue often drives the urge to grab quick, calorie-dense foods for a fast energy boost, perpetuating weight gain. Worse still, the fragmented sleep caused by apnea cuts into the deep, restorative sleep needed to keep your metabolism on track and manage your weight.

Here in the UK, a 2014 NHS report called out the lack of healthy food options available to night-shift workers in hospitals, recommending better choices in vending machines and facilities to store and reheat meals from home.[40] Sadly, ten years later, not much has changed, despite everything we know about food and diet.

So, what can you do? Here's where meal prepping and taking your own food to work can make a world of difference. Prepping your meals in advance ensures that you have healthy options ready to go, even when you're exhausted after a long shift. Instead of reaching for a sugary snack from the vending machine, you'll have something nourishing on hand that supports your health and keeps you fuelled in the right way.

If you have access to a microwave, consider meals that are easy to heat and satisfying. A protein-based hearty soup or wholegrain pasta with a simple sauce, lean protein (like grilled chicken or chickpeas) and mixed vegetables makes for a filling, nutritious option that reheats beautifully. Wholegrain wraps stuffed with hummus, grilled chicken, turkey and plenty of fresh vegetables are versatile and work well either hot or cold. For snacks, overnight oats with toppings like nuts or dried fruit, pre-portioned nuts or rice cakes with nut butter provide quick, energy-boosting options during breaks.

Although planning meals might feel like another task on your to-do list, try flipping the perspective: it's an opportunity to feel more in control and proactively address the cascade of related issues that can come from irregular eating patterns.

The unexpected shift worker

Parents often end up becoming shift workers without even realising it. Whether it's being up at all hours with a baby or, like Cassie, getting up early to stay on top of the day's chaos, it's the same grind. The difference is, no one really talks about it or sees it for what it is – a form of shift work that takes its toll. When statistics and reports talk about shift work, they usually focus on jobs like healthcare, transport, or manufacturing – roles where irregular hours are part of the deal.

But unpaid or informal roles, like parents, carers, or anyone burning the candle at both ends out of necessity, often get left out. These roles come with the same disrupted sleep, erratic eating, and stress as any formal shift work, yet the impact on their health and wellbeing rarely gets a mention. Ignoring this reality means undervaluing the physical and emotional effort that goes into these unpaid roles.

Cassie is a 36-year-old mother of two and a freelance graphic designer working from home. 'I thought working from home would make things easier,' she said. 'I could take care of the kids during the day and work at night after they went to bed.' At first, it seemed like the perfect solution – but over time, the strain of managing both began to take its toll.

'I split my workday into two shifts,' Cassie explained. 'I get up at 4 a.m. to work until the kids wake up at 7 a.m. Then, I'm a full-time mum until they go to bed around 8 p.m. After that, I work another shift until midnight or later.'

Cassie had unwittingly created a split-shift pattern that allowed her to juggle work and parenting responsibilities but meant that sleep was at the bottom of her list of priorities. 'I'm exhausted all the time,' she confessed. 'Even when I get to sleep, it doesn't feel like enough. And it's starting to affect everything – my health, my mood, my marriage.'

She described how the split-shift schedule left her feeling out of sync with her body and the rest of the world. 'I don't have a social life anymore,' she said, a note of sadness in her voice. 'I'm always too tired to go out, and even if I do, I'm thinking about the work I need to finish later.'

As Cassie spoke, it became clear that the fragmented sleep and irregular hours were taking a toll on her overall wellbeing. She was caught in a cycle of chronic sleep deprivation, compounded by the stress of trying to meet the demands of both her job and her family. 'I love my kids, and I love my work,' she said, her voice trembling slightly. 'But I don't know how much longer I can keep this up.'

'Your body needs a more consistent rhythm,' I explained. 'It's not just about getting enough sleep but about getting the right kind of sleep at the right times.' We explored the possibility of rethinking her schedule, setting clearer boundaries between work and rest, and enlisting help where possible. But with limited resources, Cassie felt these solutions were out of reach.

Her situation is a stark reflection of how societal structures often leave parents, especially mothers, bearing the brunt of impossible expectations. The lack of affordable childcare, the demands of modern work and the undervaluing of rest conspire to create unsustainable lifestyles. Cassie's story highlights a collective issue: while personal strategies are essential, addressing these pressures requires systemic change.

For now, I encouraged Cassie to take small steps within her control, like prioritising short naps or 'anchor sleep' during her best possible hours and embracing even small pockets of rest. But the truth is, we can't ignore the broader context. Stories like Cassie's should make us question why so many parents are forced into such brutal compromises – and what we, as a society, can do to change that.

How to cope with shift work

Coping with shift work is challenging for anyone and until recently, many aspects of sleep advice weren't appropriate for shift workers. These recommendations are based on a recent wide-ranging review,[41] which proposed a consensus approach to tailored guidelines to support shift workers in improving their sleep.

Prioritise sleep
- Make sleep a top priority by rescheduling social activities and household tasks.
- Inform friends, family and neighbours about your sleep schedule to minimise disruptions.
- If possible, use the anchor sleep technique from Chapter Two to guarantee a fixed period of sleep.

Aim for 7–9 hours of sleep per 24 hours
- Most healthy adults need 7–9 hours of sleep, which can be one long sleep or a main sleep plus a nap.
- Focus on total sleep time, not just time spent in bed.

Develop a sleep schedule
- Create a sleep schedule based on your work roster and lifestyle.
- Be mindful of the 'can you just' requests – protect your sleep time in the same way a non-shift worker would.
- After night shifts, consider a short sleep in the morning and go to bed earlier than usual.
- Exposure to sunlight in the morning can help realign your body clock.

Use napping as a helpful tool
- Short naps (15–20 minutes) boost alertness; longer naps (90 minutes) reduce sleep debt.

- Avoid naps longer than 20 minutes before your main sleep to prevent difficulty falling asleep.

Consider sleep inertia
- Be aware that grogginess after waking can last 15–30 minutes, up to two hours later.
- Avoid high-risk tasks like driving during this period.
- Use public transport after your shift.

Create a comfortable sleep environment
- Ensure your sleep space is cool (16–20°C/60–68°F), dark and quiet.
- Use eye masks, earplugs or white noise (if it works for you) to improve sleep quality.

Use your bed only for sleep, sickness and sex
- Avoid mentally stimulating activities in bed, like playing video games or working.
- Be mindful of pets or other disturbances in bed.

Consider light exposure
- Limit bright light exposure before bed by wearing wraparound sunglasses after night shifts until you get into bed.

Be mindful of stimulant intake
- Use caffeine to stay alert during your shift but avoid it close to bedtime as it can disrupt sleep.
- Avoid nicotine entirely or limit its use at least six hours before bed.
- Avoid using alcohol to help you fall asleep as it negatively impacts sleep quality.

Be mindful of medication
- Some medications can affect sleep; avoid stimulants before bed.

- Consult a healthcare professional regarding sleep-inducing medications or natural substances like melatonin.

Consider food intake
- Limit food intake during night shifts; opt for smaller, lighter meals if eating.
- Food prep is a valuable tool to control the food you need both at work and in the freezer for when you are too tired to cook.
- Don't go to bed hungry; choose light meals that won't cause discomfort.
- Drink enough but avoid too much fluid before bed to prevent sleep disturbances.

Engage in regular exercise
- Regular exercise supports general health and better sleep, ensuring time to cool down before bed.

Develop strategies for sleep problems
- If you can't sleep, get out of bed and do something relaxing in a quiet, dimly lit environment.
- Limit screen time and avoid clock-watching; return to bed when sleepy.
- Seek professional advice if sleep problems persist more than three times a week for several weeks.

Living in sync with time

When life feels like it's spiralling out of control, one way to rein it in is to reclaim your time and make conscious choices about how you spend it.

One way to do this is by instigating a routine. From a circadian perspective, your body will thank you for this because, at a cellular level, the body thrives on routines as the circadian system responds to and anticipates what's happening. Imagine going to bed and waking up at the same time every day. With its intricate circadian rhythm, your body will start anticipating your actions, making falling asleep and waking up easier. The pineal gland then 'knows' when to switch melatonin on and off in anticipation of bedtime and wake time.

Picture having your meals at consistent times each day. Now your digestive system, a master of routine, performs optimally with this predictability, ensuring nutrients are efficiently absorbed and blood sugar levels remain stable. Add regular timing to go to the loo, and you will start to get this well-oiled machine running well. This regularity extends to your physical activities, too. Exercise becomes not just a task but a well-timed event your body prepares for, maximising energy use and enhancing metabolic processes.

Psychologically, a routine provides a structured framework that can significantly reduce stress and anxiety. The predictability of daily activities instils a sense of control and security, alleviating the mental burden of uncertainty. Consistent sleep and wake times enhance cognitive function by ensuring the brain gets adequate rest for memory consolidation and processing. This clarity and stability contribute to better emotional regulation and overall mental wellbeing.

Socially, routines help you manage your time more efficiently, making it easier to fit in work, relaxation and social activities. Having a predictable schedule allows you to plan and enjoy social events, which can strengthen your relationships and support systems.

At a deeper biological level, your body's internal systems thrive on this routine. Hormones are released synchronously, supporting growth, appetite control and stress management. Your immune system strengthens, making you more resilient to illnesses. On a cellular level, regular sleep allows for the repair of damaged tissues, ensuring you wake up rejuvenated.

Practically, imagine winding down each night with a favourite book or a relaxing stretch and breathing session. Your body recognises these cues and starts preparing for sleep. Regular mealtimes prevent overeating and help maintain a healthy weight. Consistent exercise times enhance your physical fitness and keep your energy levels high.

But there's a middle ground to consider. When I talk about routines, remember life happens. Perfection is impossible – I prefer an 80/20 rule to give yourself some flexibility. If you think a rigid routine is the solution to all your sleep issues, you risk a slide into significant insomnia because what tends to happen is that people think it is the routine that is making them sleep, forgetting that the two processes involved in sleep (Process S and Process C, see page 17) play a significant part, as does your stress level. And there is also the reality that some people find routine difficult, if not impossible. Some people have naturally stable circadian rhythms, making establishing and sticking to routines easier. Still, others may have circadian rhythm sleep–wake disorders (CRSWD), such as delayed sleep phase disorder (DSPD), see page 243, making it difficult to maintain regular sleep and wake times. Then there are those who work shifts where routines can become problematic, if not impossible.

There is more nuance to the blue light debate

We've been told for years that bright screens before bed are terrible for our sleep.

Multiple papers suggest that melatonin levels and the time it takes to fall asleep might not be as closely linked as we once believed. The more recent research led Dr Matthew Walker to revise his stance about the blue light from screens before bed, which he had shared in his book *Why We Sleep*, and involved him admitting that he'd been too quick to warn against blue light before bedtime. The bigger issue is the activation by 'the invasion of technology into our lives and bedrooms'.[42]

The real culprit behind sleep disruption is the content itself – content engineered to hook you, to keep your attention tethered long past the point of exhaustion. Every swipe, notification and 'like' triggers a dopamine hit, the brain's reward chemical, making it difficult to disengage. It's not just stimulating your mind; it's keeping your body in a heightened state of alert, fuelled by elevated adrenaline. Your circadian rhythm isn't the only thing being disrupted – your nervous system is, too.

I cannot stress highly enough – this isn't about a lack of willpower. It isn't failure; it's manipulation. You're up against a machine – a system designed to exploit your psychological vulnerabilities. Research by James Williams, a former design ethicist at Google and PhD graduate from the Oxford Internet Institute,[43] pulls back the curtain on this manipulation, showing how digital platforms are engineered to hijack your attention by tapping into primal human desires – to be connected, informed and entertained. Tech companies profit from your attention; the longer you stay engaged, the more they gain. But you? You lose. You lose sleep, focus and the ability to consciously decide where your time should go.

With awareness comes the power to step back, recognise the game and choose differently. You don't have to play along. Reclaim your attention. Reclaim your sleep.

The next time you reach for your phone just before bed, pause. Ask yourself: Who is winning here? That moment of clarity might be all you need to break the cycle, close the app and reclaim what truly matters – your peace of mind.

Fight back

- Start by reflecting on your patterns. How often do you reach for your phone? What triggers it – boredom, stress or something deeper? Recognise these moments as opportunities to reclaim your time.
- Use technology against itself. App timers and third-party tools can help limit your social media usage. Don't rely on willpower alone – build guardrails that support your goals.
- What do you value more than another hour of scrolling? Reading, listening to music, engaging in a hobby or spending time with loved ones – these are the things that add depth and meaning to your life.

Phone overuse, especially at night, isn't just about boredom or habit. Often, something deeper drives it – a need for control or avoidance. An often overlooked factor is perfectionism.

Perfectionism doesn't just show up at work or in creative projects; it seeps into daily life. The need to be 'on top' of everything – to respond to messages immediately, end the day with an empty mailbox, resolve every conversation and be constantly available – becomes a silent burden. The device becomes a way to manage all of it. But I find that often, this compulsion isn't just being connected; it's about feeling like you've done enough, that you're still productive and engaged, even when the rest of the world is winding down. Stopping and letting go – even for the necessity of sleep – can trigger anxiety. The mind races, questioning whether you've done enough today, whether you've missed something, whether you're falling behind. The device becomes both a distraction from that discomfort and its source. The result? A spiral of stress and stimulation that makes sleep increasingly elusive.

Always 'on'

You might be surprised at how often I see this as a key driver for insomnia; it reflects a culture that equates busyness with worth. We're pushed to do more, achieve more and prove more, often at the expense of our wellbeing. Stepping away from that narrative can feel like swimming upstream.

Linked closely to perfectionism is the need to always feel valuable and necessary. It's the belief that your worth is measured by your productivity – by how much you do or control. This drive can manifest as a compulsion to fill every moment, avoiding stillness at all costs. After all, if you're not doing something, are you still valuable?

When this drive becomes ingrained, even the act of resting feels uncomfortable. It's as if time is slipping through your fingers and you're letting yourself down by not doing enough. But this discomfort isn't entirely your fault; it's a response to a culture that values doing over being, productivity over peace. And so, in moments of unease, you reach for something – anything – to fill the void. However, what begins as a coping mechanism only deepens the problem. Despite all this activity, the anxiety lingers, and sleep, once your body's natural refuge, slips further out of reach.

This struggle manifests differently for different people, each with a unique approach to routine, yet all driven by similar underlying fears and desires.

When we explore our relationship with time, we are also delving into how we've been conditioned to meet the expectations we believe others have of us. This conditioning begins in childhood and is shaped by the standards our caregivers set for us. Perhaps you had a high-achieving parent who, with the best intentions, set a standard you felt compelled to meet. Or maybe you rebelled against it, creating a different kind of tension within yourself. Either way, the pressure to conform or resist can create stress that seeps into your relationship with time, routine and, by default, sleep.

One way to cope with overwhelming stress or anxiety is to try to take control of the situation – to try harder. This instinct makes sense – it's natural to want to regain a sense of stability when life feels chaotic. However, this need for control can become increasingly rigid and intense over time, leading to a cycle where the drive for control tightens its grip. This often manifests as perfectionism – a common but sometimes harmful response to the pressures we feel both within ourselves and from the expectations of others. It's an unconscious survival strategy that begins in our earliest years.

As we grow, this need evolves into something more complex: the drive to belong, to fit in, to be perfect in the eyes of others. Perfectionism whispers, 'If I can just get everything right, then I will be safe.' But this pursuit of perfection often backfires, especially when it comes to something as natural as sleep. It can propel us to achieve great things but frequently leaves us wondering, 'When will I be enough?'

It can be deeply uncomfortable to dig into the roots of our perfectionism, to face the possibility that much of our striving is driven by a fear of inadequacy. The more we crave control, the more rigid and brittle we become, and the more afraid we are of what will happen if we let go.

What would it mean to you to let go of the need to have everything perfectly planned and just let life unfold? Could you embrace the messiness, the uncertainty, and trust yourself to handle whatever comes your way? In those moments of not knowing, there's a chance to find a deeper kind of peace – one that isn't tied to everything going exactly as you'd imagined.

It's OK to let go. If you can find a way to a place of 'enough is enough', you might find the rest and relaxation you've been craving.

Summary

How you manage time affects your health, happiness and fulfilment; life's constant demands can clash with your body's needs, leading to stress and sleep issues. Accept that time is finite and precious. This realisation can bring profound meaning and help you prioritise what's truly important. Regain control by slowing down and living intentionally. It's time to say 'no' to the tech giants who design attention-grabbing apps, 'no' to back-to-back Zoom meetings and 'no' to staying inside all day.

Try to take the time to sit on your doorstep or by an open window with your morning coffee or spend more time outside during your commute. Consider walking meetings or taking non-smoking breaks during the day.

By making small adjustments and tuning in to your chronotype – working during your peak productivity, socialising when you're most engaged and giving rest the attention it deserves – you can boost your wellbeing and create a more natural flow in your daily life.

Decide deliberately how to spend your time. Cut out non-essential activities and focus on what brings value and joy to your life. Lower stress levels improve sleep and make you feel more relaxed and in control.

This sets the stage for the next chapter on managing stress. Time is finite, a constant reminder of our mortality. Yet, this limitation holds the potential for profound meaning and connection. Embracing natural rhythms and making mindful choices about your time allow you to live more fully and authentically. Living this way reduces stress, improves health and enhances happiness. Relationships deepen as you become more present and engaged, free from rushed schedules – perhaps it's a utopian dream, but change is possible if we all take steps towards it.

Actionable steps

- Understand that time is finite and invaluable; avoid letting others dictate it.
- Identify and mitigate activities that create time poverty, like overworking and sacrificing rest.

- Acknowledge and incorporate various types of rest: physical, mental, sensory, creative, emotional, social and spiritual.
- Understand circadian rhythms and their regulation by the suprachiasmatic nucleus.
- Discover your chronotype (morning larks, intermediate types, night owls) and how that works for you.
- Maintain a consistent sleep schedule to improve health and longevity.
- Have a protein-based breakfast at the same time every day.
- Recognise the inefficiency of multitasking and focus on single tasking.
- Explore and integrate different forms of rest into daily routines.
- Increase natural light exposure during the day and put the devices away in the evening.
- If you're a shift worker, consider what steps you can take to prioritise your sleep and health.
- Manage screen time effectively and prioritise pre-bedtime relaxation.
- Use time cues (meal timing, social interactions, physical activity) to synchronise biological clocks.
- Address the psychological impacts of digital communication and prioritise genuine connections.
- Pick a few key activities – like waking up, eating or winding down for bed – and commit to doing them at the same time every day. Consistency helps these actions become automatic, reducing mental effort and stress while strengthening your body's natural rhythm. Start small, stay consistent and let the benefits build over time.

CHAPTER FIVE

Untangling the relationship between stress and sleep

Stress and sleep are two deeply intertwined aspects of our lives. Together, they are two ends of an invisible thread stretched taut – life's demands pulling on one end, the biological need for sleep tugging on the other. Zina's relentless work schedule, Alex's constant pressures and Ivan's struggles with shifting priorities. If you've ever found yourself staring at the ceiling, unable to drift off no matter how tired you are, you're not alone. Stress can hijack even the most exhausted mind. But what exactly is happening in your body and brain when stress prevents you from resting?

The answer lies in the autonomic nervous system (ANS) – your body's autopilot. Quietly and constantly, the ANS manages vital functions like your heartbeat, breathing and digestion without any conscious effort. Its primary job is to keep you safe, scanning your environment and asking the critical question: *Am I safe?*

When the ANS detects danger, it activates the fight-or-flight response to protect you. Imagine you're walking down the street, lost in thought, when you step into traffic. In that split second, your body reacts faster than your conscious mind. Your ANS leaps into action, triggering the release of adrenaline and cortisol. Adrenaline provides an immediate burst of energy, sharpening your reflexes and heightening your senses to help you react quickly. Cortisol, often called the 'stress hormone', sustains this heightened state, keeping you alert and focused until the danger has passed. These hormones work together to protect you, ensuring you survive the moment before you even have time to think.

This ancient system evolved to save us from immediate dangers like predators or accidents. It's designed to keep you awake and alert when survival is at stake. But in today's world, this same mechanism often misfires. Your body reacts to modern stressors – an email notification, a looming deadline or a tense conversation – as though they were life-threatening.

Flipping the script on stress

It's easy to view stress as a weakness, a flaw or something to be avoided. Many of us label stress as a failure or a sign that we aren't coping well enough. I recall a friend's frustration when their doctor attributed their symptoms to stress. 'How could *that* be causing *all this*?' they demanded.

What if you could lean into stress instead of resisting it? What if you saw stress not as a threat, but as a signal? Stress isn't a sign of weakness – it's your body's way of saying, *Something here matters. Pay attention.*

When you consciously notice stress, it can become a teacher, showing you what you care about most. By approaching it with curiosity instead of resistance, you can reframe stress as your fiercest protector. You don't need to 'get rid of stress'; you need to work with it and hear its need.

The next time stress keeps you awake, try this instead:

- **Pause.** Check in with yourself: *Am I safe?*
- **Reframe.** Ask: *What is my body trying to protect me from?*
- **Support.** What do I need right now to feel safe and calm?

By calming your stress response – letting it know you are safe – you create the conditions for restful sleep. Stress becomes your silent protector, working with you rather than against you.

Allostasis – the body will always balance the books

When stress hits, your body enters a state of allostasis – balancing short-term survival needs against long-term health. This prioritisation doesn't always feel good. For example, in fight-or-flight mode your body uses up energy faster and takes in less, like getting less oxygen. Quick, shallow breaths are less efficient at oxygen exchange compared with deep, slow breaths. This means you might take in less oxygen despite breathing faster, which can lead to feelings of light-headedness or shortness of breath. In shutdown mode, it saves energy. It also 'braces' for impact, tightening all the muscles leading to distorted tension – think headaches and back and shoulder pain.

These responses have evolved to help us manage our limited resources effectively. Imagine your hormones, brain chemicals and nerve pathways working together to keep you functioning. Under normal circumstances, this system helps you shift smoothly between states of alertness and relaxation throughout the day. However, when this system gets disrupted, it affects more than just your mood – you might find yourself feeling constantly stressed or emotionally numb and detached. This disruption also impacts sleep. In fight-or-flight mode, your body is too tense to relax, making it difficult to fall or stay asleep. On the flip side, if you're stuck in shutdown mode, you might sleep excessively but still wake up exhausted.[1]

Cortisol: what you need to know

Cortisol is a steroid hormone produced by the adrenal glands, located just above the kidneys. Often called the 'stress hormone', it has multiple roles, including regulating metabolism, supporting immune function and managing the sleep–wake cycle. Essentially, it powers the body's response to stress.

Cortisol and sleep

Cortisol doesn't just react to stress; it also follows a daily pattern called the cortisol awakening response (CAR). It peaks in the early morning to help you wake up and gradually declines throughout the day to promote sleep at night. This morning surge makes you feel alert and energised, preparing you for the day ahead.

Cortisol and melatonin – the hormone that promotes sleep – work together in a hormonal dance, influencing the other's levels. About 12 to 14 hours after cortisol peaks in the morning, your pineal gland starts to produce melatonin – signalling to your body that it's time to wind down and prepare for sleep.

- **Top tip:** Getting up, going outside and moving first thing in the morning can positively influence your hormonal balance, positively affecting cortisol and melatonin levels. Gentle morning activity, like walking outside, can enhance alertness and energy levels by supporting cortisol's role in mobilising energy stores, without overstimulating the stress response. Morning light, especially from the blue spectrum, signals to your brain's suprachiasmatic nucleus (SCN) to regulate the sleep–wake cycle.

Persistently elevated cortisol levels may suppress melatonin production, interfering with your ability to fall and stay asleep. Paradoxically, over time, your body might respond to prolonged high cortisol by reducing its production, leading to abnormally low levels. This reduced cortisol response can cause daytime fatigue and still not improve sleep disturbances, demonstrating how both excessively high and low cortisol levels cause problems.

Baseline cortisol levels, as well as the body's response to stress, vary widely from person to person. These differences are influenced by factors like genetics, early life experiences, current stressors and certain medical conditions. Because of this, what helps regulate cortisol for one person may not work as well for another.

The risks of over-focusing on one issue

In the quest to manage stress and improve wellbeing, cortisol is often singled out as the root cause of numerous health issues. While it plays a key role in stress and sleep regulation, it's just one part of a complex system involving diet, sleep, exercise and emotional health. Simplistic approaches marketed to 'fix cortisol' often lack scientific basis and can increase anxiety by overemphasising a single factor. Instead, recognise the complexity of your physiology and seek personalised advice from a healthcare professional to make informed, balanced choices for your health.

The autonomic nervous system and your emotional world

As you move down the ladder, you enter what's known as the 'fight-or-flight' system – the part of your nervous system that kicks in when your body senses danger. It's like your internal alarm system, putting you on high alert to keep you safe. When this happens, a lot of changes start to take place in your body: your heart beats faster to send more blood to your muscles, giving you the energy to fight or run; your focus locks onto the threat, so you're less aware of anything else; your muscles tense up, which can leave you feeling stiff or even shaky.

You might notice your digestion slows down – leading to that fluttery, nauseous feeling in your stomach – or, depending on the situation, you might urgently need the loo or experience constipation as your body 'holds on'. While this state is crucial in emergencies, staying here too long can leave you feeling stuck on edge, making it really hard to relax or sleep. Your body is ready for action, not rest, and it takes effort to climb back up the ladder to a calm and safe state.

The autonomic nervous system (ANS) is deeply tied to your emotions, as it's designed to ensure survival. During emotional conflicts, such as arguments, your body may interpret the intensity as danger, activating a stress response. This only eases when the ANS detects safety, allowing you to relax and sleep.

Traditionally, we think of the ANS as having two parts: the sympathetic nervous system (SNS) and the parasympathetic nervous system (PNS). The SNS is activated in response to stress, leading to the 'fight-or-flight' response, which increases heart rate and breathing, and mobilises energy to act.

The PNS promotes 'rest-and-digest' functions, helping the body to relax and recover. It slows down the heart rate and aids digestion, making sleeping easier.

Polyvagal theory (PVT), devised by Dr Stephen Porges, explains how your nervous system responds to the world around you, influencing how safe or stressed you feel.[2] Why does this matter for sleep? First, because your body needs to feel safe to truly relax and let you drift off and second, these states carry over into sleep. Deb Dana, who has been a pioneer in applying PVT to the practice of psychotherapy, took this idea and created a simple 'ladder' analogy to bring it to life.[3] Each rung represents a different state of mind and body, showing how you can move between feeling calm and connected, ready to fight or flee, or completely shut down. It's a useful way to think about how you respond to life's challenges and also to know that you move between these states (important if you are depressed or anxious).

Calm and connected (top of the ladder)

This is your 'safe zone'. You feel relaxed, grounded and secure. Your heart rate is steady, your digestion works smoothly and you feel open to connecting with others. Sleep in this state is easy and restorative, helping your body and mind recharge.

If you're stuck in stress or overwhelm, it's harder to access this state, which can lead to insomnia. Your body needs to feel calm and safe for sleep to come naturally.

Alert and reactive (middle of the ladder)

This is your fight-or-flight state – your body's alarm system for dealing with stress or danger. Your heart beats faster, your muscles tense and digestion slows down to save energy for action.

How this might feel? Anxious, restless or hyper-focused. Your thoughts might race and your body feels like it's constantly 'on'. Tension in the body builds up and gets expressed through muscle activity like jaw clenching (bruxism) or teeth grinding.

What happens to sleep? Your nervous system is primed for action, not rest. Even if you're tired, your body won't let its guard down enough for you to fall or stay asleep, as well as keeping you in light sleep for most of the night so you wake up exhausted.

Associated sleep disorders: insomnia is common here, as is restless legs syndrome (RLS), where stress can make your body feel too restless to relax.

Shutdown and disconnected (bottom of the ladder)

When stress feels too overwhelming, your body might switch into shutdown mode. It's like hitting the brakes hard to conserve energy. You might feel numb, hopeless or completely drained.

How this might feel? Everything slows down – you might feel heavy, detached or stuck. Digestion often grinds to a halt, leading to bloating or constipation.

What happens to sleep? Because the body is in energy conservation mode, not the calm state needed for true recovery, you might find yourself sleeping for longer but it's not restorative.

Associated sleep disorders: Hypersomnia (excessive sleep) can happen here, as can sleep disturbances like apnea or parasomnias (like night terrors).

Your nervous system is designed to adapt, shifting between these states depending on what's going on. For example, you might feel calm and connected while spending time with friends, shift into fight-or-flight when stressed, and then need a nap to recover if it all becomes too much.

The problem arises when you get stuck — whether it's in the hyperactive middle state (fight-or-flight) or the low-energy bottom state (shutdown). Chronic stress, overwhelm, or trauma can keep your nervous system from resetting, leaving you feeling constantly "on" or drained.

You can help your nervous system climb back to the top of the ladder with simple steps:

For fight-or-flight (middle of the ladder):
- Try deep breathing to slow your heart rate and calm your body.
- Progressive muscle relaxation can ease tension in your muscles.
- Grounding exercises, like focusing on your senses, can help bring you back to the present moment.

For shutdown (bottom of the ladder):
- Gentle movement, like stretching, gentle walking or yoga, can help re-engage your body.
- Connecting with someone safe can help you feel less isolated.
- Small, manageable tasks can help build momentum and a sense of energy.

You can also experience combinations of these states, which helps you recognise that your stress responses are complex and can vary depending on the situation. It's not always just about being calm, ready to fight or run, or completely shut down; you can experience a blend of these responses simultaneously, affecting how you experience the world. A panic attack is a classic example of when fight-or-flight and shutdown are present simultaneously and create freeze. There is a huge amount of energy in the system, but it is unable to be discharged.

Understanding where you are on this ladder at any given moment helps you make sense of your reactions and makes sense of the tools you need to help you to move back up towards safety and connection.

The goal isn't to keep you permanently calm and relaxed – life just doesn't work that way. Instead, it's about helping you move smoothly between different emotional states without getting stuck, especially in high-stress states like fight-or-flight or complete shutdown. The aim is to build your emotional flexibility, so you can respond to what's happening around you without feeling overwhelmed.

A big part of this is learning to use something called the 'vagal brake'.[4] Think of it as a brake that can slow down your heart, helping you stay calm when you need to. When the brake is on, your heart rate slows, making it easier to feel relaxed. When the brake is off, your heart rate speeds up, preparing you to deal with stress or danger.

Imagine you're about to give a big presentation, and the nerves kick in – your heart races and your hands feel shaky. Keep it simple: use your breath to steady yourself. Inhale for a count of four, five or six, and exhale for the same count. This balanced breathing activates your vagus nerve, applying the 'brake' to your stress response. As your heart rate slows, you'll feel more grounded, calm and ready to take on the challenge. Think of the vagal brake as your body's built-in stress regulator – it helps you stay calm and focused when it matters most. By understanding how your nervous system constantly shifts gears throughout the day, you can see how these adjustments impact your ability to unwind and sleep at night.

Where are you right now? – triggers and glimmers

The word 'triggered' has become part of everyday language, often used to describe moments of stress, upset or emotional overwhelm. In its truest sense, a trigger is something that pulls you down the nervous system ladder into states of stress or shutdown. It could lead to feelings like panic, anxiety or sadness, and physical reactions such as a racing heart, tense muscles, or even a sense of numbness or disconnection. Triggers are often tied to past experiences of stress or trauma, and they can leave you feeling stuck in fight-or-flight or completely immobilised.

While recognising triggers is important, the conversation can sometimes feel heavily focused on what pulls us down. That's where the idea of glimmers, again introduced by Deb Dana, brings balance and hope. Glimmers are the small, positive moments that pull you up the ladder, back towards a state of calm, safety and connection. These might be as simple as the sound of birds singing, the warmth of the sun on your skin or the comforting purr of your cat. It's so easy to get caught up in the 'bad stuff – we're all wired with a natural negativity bias, after all. That's why it's worth reminding yourself to stop and notice the good. Take a moment to pause and look for the little things that glimmer in your life. On a day when everything feels like it's going wrong (and you haven't slept), maybe the only good thing is that it's not raining. But hey, that's still something! Even on the tough days, there's always a little bit of good if you're willing to spot it.

I am all too aware that at times life is truly unbearable. Let's be clear: glimmers don't erase the pain, and they're not some cure-all for the weight of life's challenges. But they are something real – a flicker of relief, a moment of light in the darkness. They won't fix everything, but they can remind you that even in the worst moments, there's still something to hold onto, something that says, 'You're still here.' And sometimes, that's enough to keep going.

In his 2013 TED Talk, Dr Rick Hanson describes this as 'building islands in the stream'.[5] By intentionally noticing and savouring small, positive moments, you create tiny pockets of stability and strength in the flow of life. These 'islands' may seem small, but over time they create a foundation for resilience and a sense of wellbeing that can help you navigate even the hardest times.

These micro-moments can also strengthen your vagal brake – the part of your nervous system that helps you manage stress and stay balanced. Both triggers and glimmers influence how you move up and down the nervous system ladder. Triggers pull you into states of stress and overwhelm, while glimmers help you climb back towards calm and connection. As a psychotherapist, I'd say that just knowing what your triggers are and how to handle them is one of the most valuable things you can do for yourself. Triggers can pull you into stress or shutdown, but understanding what sets them off gives you a sense of control and clarity. It's not about avoiding them completely – that's not realistic – but when you know what's happening, you can start to make space for a pause, ground yourself and respond in a way that feels manageable.

Recognising glimmers doesn't mean ignoring the reality of triggers, but it reminds us to also notice the small joys and moments of safety that are still there, waiting to be appreciated.

How to notice your triggers and collect glimmers

Triggers

Pay attention to your body – do you notice tension, a racing heart or a knot in your stomach?

Reflect on patterns – are there situations, places, or interactions that often leave you feeling stressed or overwhelmed?

Write them down to build awareness and start recognising early signs.

Glimmers

Keep a list of small moments that make you feel calm or safe, like a favourite song, a scent you love or watching the clouds.

Pause during the day to notice when you feel even a little bit of joy or peace, and make a mental note.

Use your glimmers during stressful moments as reminders that safety and calm are still within reach.

By noticing and appreciating glimmers, you're doing more than just enjoying fleeting moments of positivity – you're actively turning down the stress dial, training your brain to feel calmer and setting yourself up for a better night's sleep.

A gentle reminder

We often blame poor sleep for exhaustion and lack of focus, but chronic stress is usually the real culprit. Understanding this is the first step to breaking out of survival mode. But there's another layer to consider: that inner voice, the one that tends to be your harshest critic. While stress affects your body, this internal dialogue can take a toll on your mind, making it even harder to recover and find balance. Recognising both is key to moving forward.

Can you treat yourself with the same kindness you offer others? Think about it – would you speak to a friend or loved one the way you sometimes speak to yourself? Probably not. When someone you care about is struggling, you'd likely offer a kind word, a hug or a reassuring gesture. You can activate your own 'caregiving system' in the same way. This releases oxytocin, a hormone that benefits your heart and helps reduce anxiety, especially the kind tied to stress, burnout and survival mode.

If showing yourself that same kindness feels difficult, it might be worth exploring in therapy. Your inner voice didn't appear out of nowhere – it's learned. Understanding where it came from and learning to quiet it can be a transformative step towards healing and balance. After all, treating yourself with compassion isn't just a nice idea – it's a powerful way to begin breaking free from the stress cycle.

The many faces of stress and sleep

Hyperarousal: Perry's insomnia

Perry didn't believe he was stressed – until he started paying attention. The previous week, I had introduced the ladder analogy from polyvagal theory and asked him to track his emotional states using an emotional tracker. Now, sitting across from me, shoulders slumped, he shared his realisation: 'Now that I'm noticing how I feel, my stress is off the scale.'

This admission was heavy but vital – he was beginning to bridge the gap between how he felt and how he thought he should feel. 'It's like I have this scorpion inside me,' he said, 'always ready to strike – at anything.' The analogy captured the hyperarousal driving his severe insomnia. How could anyone sleep with a scorpion, ready to attack at the slightest trigger?

I explained how his body and mind were in constant overdrive, bracing for something to go wrong. In this state, his muscles stayed tense – just like the scorpion he described, always poised to strike.

No wonder Perry felt overwhelmed. 'It's like I can never relax, never let my guard down,' he said.

I reflected on its presence, observing that it was a part of him but not all of him. He was stuck in the fight-or-flight zone of the SNS. It was a response, a protective mechanism that had perhaps been overactivated. I asked him what he thought it was protecting him from. He frowned, considering this. 'I don't know . . . maybe failure, maybe just . . . life. I've always felt like I had to be on top of everything, like if I slipped up, everything would fall apart.'

So many of us have internalised the fear of failure. Understanding that your fear of failure is closely linked to a fear of losing safety and security can help you address the root causes of this fear.

I asked if he could remember moments when he felt calm and happy, even from long ago. They might serve as a reminder that it's possible to feel that way again. In a previous session, he had mentioned a love of architecture, so I asked if he could find safe places or activities that would allow him to reconnect with that love.

For Perry, small levers were the way forward. As he reflected, he realised that taking a lunchtime walk to admire the buildings around him – or, if he couldn't get outside, looking at architecture photos online – could

Perry's emotional tracker

(notice that he added a scorpion to represent hyperarousal and used a mixture of emojis)

Date	Happiness 🙂	Sadness 🙁	Anger 😠	Fear 😨	Stress 😣	Hyperarousal 🦂	Notes
1		🙁		😨	😣	🦂	
2	🙂	🙁	😠	😨	😣	😝	
3		🙁	😠	😨	😣	😝	
...							
29		🙁	😠	😨	😣	😝	
30	🙂			😨	😣	😝	
31				😨	😣	😝	

help him reconnect with a sense of calm. We also discussed adding simple breathing techniques to give him a tool for slowing down in the moment.

Did Perry's sleep improve? Gradually, yes. The scorpion on high alert didn't disappear overnight, but its grip started to loosen. His progress was steady, proof that even small steps can lead to meaningful change.

Create your own emotion tracker

I devised the emotion tracker template on page 158 and use it in my work with clients, but for this book, I've created an example inspired by 'Perry', a fictional construct designed to show how the tool can work in real life while maintaining confidentiality. You can use this template as it is or adapt it to fit your own style. Adding emojis or colours to represent emotions makes it visually engaging and helps you map your emotional landscape more clearly.

Some people track their emotions once a day, while others break it down further, adding columns for morning, afternoon and evening to capture fluctuations. Over time, this builds a record that might surprise you. For instance, you may look back on what felt like a non-stop stressful month and find that your own evidence – your happiness indicators – tell a different story. It's a simple but powerful way to gain insight, balance your perspective and connect with your emotional patterns.

Hypoarousal: Clary's hypersomnia

Unlike Perry, whose stress kept him awake, Clary's stress pushed her into shutdown. As a high school teacher and mother of three, Clary was once the embodiment of 'organised chaos'. She thrived amid the bustling demands of her life, moving seamlessly from managing a classroom full of teenagers to orchestrating her children's lives. But post-pandemic, that energy and enthusiasm began to wither. Overwhelmed by years of caregiving and self-sacrifice, she began sleeping excessively during the day, feeling disconnected and unrefreshed.

When she finally sought help, Clary was diagnosed with depression and hypersomnia, a chronic and often debilitating condition marked by excessive daytime sleepiness that doesn't improve with rest (see page 228). While many are familiar with insomnia, hypersomnia often goes unnoticed, though its impact can be considerably debilitating.

In our sessions, we identified her state as hypoarousal – a kind of shutdown where the body, overwhelmed by exhaustion, essentially shuts down to survive. 'Your body is trying to conserve energy,' I explained. 'It's saying, "I can't keep up with this pace anymore."' But understanding this wasn't enough; we needed to find ways for Clary to reconnect with life and climb out of this state of withdrawal.[6]

As we explored her story, a buried memory surfaced. At ten years old, Clary's life changed when her mother fell seriously ill. As the eldest of four children, she became the caretaker, managing the household with a sense of duty far beyond her years. Her father, overwhelmed, leaned on her heavily. There was no space for her to express fear, exhaustion or vulnerability.

This experience left a lasting mark. Clary grew into adulthood believing her worth was tied to her ability to manage everything, care for others and maintain control – no matter the cost to herself. But now, decades later, that unspoken contract was breaking down.

Navigating shame and the need for rest

One of Clary's biggest hurdles was her guilt and shame about needing extra rest. 'How do I explain that I need to take regular naps?' she asked, frustrated. 'It feels like I'm making excuses, but if I push through, the exhaustion multiplies to the point where I don't even recognise myself anymore.'

Her secret naps at school caused constant anxiety. She worried that her colleagues or students would judge her as unprofessional or incapable, and hiding her need for rest only reinforced her shame. Clary's struggle wasn't just practical; it stemmed from deep-seated beliefs about what it meant to be strong, capable and worthy. Like many women, she had internalised the message that a 'good' mother, professional or person handles everything without complaint or rest. Asking for accommodations felt like betraying those expectations.

Together, we worked to reframe her thoughts using cognitive-behavioural techniques and self-compassion exercises. I reminded her that needing rest didn't make her weak – it made her human. 'Your body isn't betraying you,' I explained. 'It's protecting you in the only way it knows how.'

Creating a positive relationship with napping

Together, we brainstormed practical solutions to establish a positive nap structure that she could manage as a matter of course. Clary realised that making her naps a regular, acknowledged part of her day could alleviate much of the shame and secrecy that weighed her down.

We explored how Clary could come to terms with and normalise taking rest and napping as a regular, supportive part of her day – something she could rely on without guilt or secrecy. By creating a gentle, practical structure around her need for rest, Clary began to release the shame that had been weighing her down and instead see this as an act of care for herself.

The next step was implementing this in her workplace, but taking that step wasn't easy. Clary felt significant anxiety about approaching her supervisor to discuss her needs. Disclosing a chronic medical condition at work is more than just a personal challenge – it carries very real risks. Across workplaces worldwide, such disclosures can sometimes lead to stigma, discrimination or even job loss. The fear of being judged, overlooked for opportunities or penalised often makes staying silent feel like the safer option.

Despite these concerns, Clary found the courage to have an open and honest conversation with her supervisor. She explained her condition and how a brief, scheduled nap could enhance her productivity and wellbeing. To her relief, her supervisor was not only understanding but also supportive, collaborating with her to implement the adjustments she needed.

The school agreed to provide a quiet, private space where Clary could take her naps. This eliminated the need to hide and reduced her anxiety about being discovered. She incorporated her naps into her daily schedule, treating them with the same importance as any other professional responsibility. This helped normalise the practice for herself and those around her.

She began to practise mindfulness and self-compassion exercises, reminding herself that taking care of her needs was not selfish but necessary. Over time, Clary began to climb out of the depths of hypoarousal. It wasn't an overnight transformation – such things rarely are. But with each small step, she started to reclaim parts of herself that had been lost to exhaustion.

In our final sessions, Clary reflected on her progress. 'I still have days where I feel like I'm drowning,' she admitted, 'but I can see that's where I am – I am not lost in it anymore. I also have days where I can see the shore. I'm starting to feel more like myself again and learning that it's OK to ask for help when I need it.'

Sadly, Clary's experience underscores the immense bravery it can take to seek support, whether from others or in the workplace. Managing a chronic health condition or disability is often intertwined with challenges like disrupted sleep and mental health struggles, making the process even more complex.

Napping on the job

I often ask people: 'Does your workplace support napping?' The answer is almost always no. Responses vary – some laugh as if it's absurd, others express anxiety about sleeping at their desk, and many fear being judged as lazy. This reflects a persistent myth: that taking a break, let alone napping, is unproductive.

Science, however, tells a different story. Research consistently shows that well-timed naps boost alertness, creativity and productivity. Companies like Google have embraced nap pods because of these proven benefits. Yet, the stigma persists. Our 'presenteeism' culture prioritises long hours and constant busyness over meaningful results, viewing rest as indulgent or weak.

Take night-shift workers, for example. Studies show that naps during shifts improve alertness and performance, even though the benefits are limited compared with full night-time sleep.[7] A study on factory workers found that longer naps during night shifts (from 1 a.m. to 3 a.m. or 3 a.m. to 5 a.m.) reduced sleepiness at the end of the shift, although the workers still felt much more tired compared with how they felt after sleeping during the day.[8] Even so, that slight improvement in alertness could significantly affect performance and safety.

It's likely that practical barriers like busy schedules, lack of quiet spaces or fear of judgement often prevent them. Sleep inertia, or post-nap grogginess, is another challenge, particularly at night, which is why a recovery window of 15–30 minutes is critical before returning to high-stakes tasks.[9]

So why hasn't the workplace embraced naps? The science is clear, but outdated ideas about productivity hold us back. It's time to rethink our values: should we prioritise appearances of busyness, or invest in evidence-based strategies like strategic rest to deliver high-quality, meaningful work?

Mastering naptime

Napping at the right time can be incredibly refreshing, even if you don't fall asleep – just resting helps. Letting go of the pressure to sleep allows you to naturally slip into lighter sleep stages, like N1 and N2, which can still be restorative. However, timing is key. Poorly timed naps can lead to sleep inertia. Your brain needs a few minutes to fully reboot before performing at its best, so always build in recovery time after a nap.[10]

About napping

The short nap (power nap)
- **Duration:** a brief, refreshing 20–30 minutes.
- **When:** early afternoon, ideally between 1 p.m. and 3 p.m., or during a suitable break in your shift.
- **Benefits:** this short nap keeps you in the lighter stages of non-REM sleep, avoiding the depths of deep sleep. It's akin to a quick interlude in your day, offering you a burst of energy and clarity without the grogginess caused by sleep inertia.

The longer nap (part of biphasic sleep)
- **Duration:** a complete sleep cycle, 90–120 minutes.
- **When:** mid-afternoon, around 2 p.m. to 4 p.m.
- **Benefits:** this nap embraces an entire sleep cycle, traversing light sleep, deep sleep and REM sleep. It's perfect if you're following a biphasic sleep pattern, where your rest is divided into two phases – one main period at night and a shorter, revitalising nap during the day.

Avoiding the pitfall of sleep inertia

For short naps:

- **Set a non-alarming alarm:** ensure your nap remains brief, not extending beyond 20–30 minutes, to prevent you from descending into a deep sleep, where waking becomes harder and sleep inertia lurks.
- **Create a sanctuary:** find a quiet, dark place to nap. If it works for you, an eye mask or earplugs can help you to drop out of your environment, allowing you to relax fully.

For longer naps:

- **Embrace the full cycle:** a 90–120-minute nap allows your body to experience a complete sleep cycle, reducing the risk of waking from deep sleep and the accompanying grogginess.
- **Protect your nightly sleep:** if you have insomnia or find it hard to maintain a solid block of sleep at night, avoid these longer naps. You don't want to spend any of your hard-earned sleep pressure disrupting your night-time rest.

General tips for the perfect nap:

- **Listen to your body:** tune in to your natural rhythms, recognising when your body needs rest.
- **Keep a consistent schedule:** regularity can help regulate your body clock, making your naps more restorative.
- **Avoid late-afternoon naps or napping within six hours of your main sleep:** napping too late can intrude upon your overall sleep, particularly if insomnia is a challenge.

Differentiating between acute and chronic stress, little-'t' trauma and big-'T' trauma

In these turbulent times, it's unsurprising that many of us are reaching breaking point. If there were ever an example of the importance of feeling safe and what happens when we don't, the pandemic showed us.

The trials of the pandemic have tested our resilience, and it's clear that post-pandemic, the stress of our modern world is pushing us to the edge. I continue to be amazed that it happened, and yet society seems to have pushed it under the metaphorical rug, as though we can just carry on as usual. This phenomenon is not new; societies have faced similar struggles throughout history. Today, however, there is a more profound understanding of the physiological and psychological impacts of stress and trauma, yet society still refuses to act to mitigate these effects.

When the autonomic nervous system (ANS) is pushed beyond its limits, it enters the realm of trauma. Gabor Maté, a physician and author known for his work on addiction, stress and childhood development, provides a compelling definition of trauma: that it is not about the events that happen to us but about how we internally process and experience them. It's about the emotional and psychological imprints they leave behind, often disconnecting us from ourselves, others and our environment, thereby affecting our ability to be fully present.[11] There's an ongoing discussion about whether stress or trauma has a more profound impact on our wellbeing. Psychiatrist Judith Herman's groundbreaking work offers further clarity. She makes use of the concepts of big-T and little-t trauma.[12]

Big-T traumas are the major, life-altering events we all recognise – the loss of a parent, child or spouse; natural disasters; wars; severe accidents. These events often have immediate and overwhelming psychological impacts, shaking the very foundation of our sense of safety and stability.

Little-t traumas, on the other hand, are the subtler, often overlooked experiences – the chronic stress of caring for an ailing loved one, enduring repeated emotional neglect or navigating the slow erosion of trust in a relationship. While these might not cause an immediate breakdown, their cumulative weight can profoundly influence our mental health, leaving us less equipped to manage stress over time.

Both types of trauma matter. The human experience is complex, and our responses to these events – big or small – shape how we navigate life's challenges.

Mixed states: Damian's frozen fight

Damian's experience reflected a clash between hyperarousal and hypoarousal. 'I'm stuck between two states,' he said, describing how his mind raced while his body felt immobilised. He entered my office like a man under siege – eyes darting, shoulders slumped and restlessness spilling out as he spoke. 'I feel like I'm racing against something I can't see. My body feels like it's betraying me – gut pain, exhaustion, no sleep. It's like my body is sending me a message I can't decode.'

Damian's words reflected a state I often see in my clients – what I call 'frantic inertia'. It's like his body was a car with both the accelerator and brake pressed down at the same time. The accelerator – the stress response – kept him on high alert, constantly ready to react, while the brake – the shutdown response – tried to conserve energy. The result? He was stuck, revving internally but unable to move forward or fully stop and rest.

When I asked him, 'Do you feel safe?' he gave me a look of disbelief. 'Safe?' he repeated, almost laughing. 'At work? No one's safe. It's cut-throat. You've got to watch your back every second.' Damian's nervous system had adapted to an environment where safety wasn't an option, leaving him trapped in this exhausting state of push-and-pull. It was clear that his feelings of unsafety at work were part of a bigger picture, one we needed to understand to help him move forward.

In our next session, something shifted. As he paced the room, Damian began reflecting on his past. 'It's not just work,' he admitted, his voice quieter now. 'The boys at school . . . they used to torment me. I never felt safe – not for a single day.' As he spoke, his hand drifted to his stomach, where he had long felt pain. 'It's fear,' he realised. 'Fear that's been sitting there for years.'[13]

This revelation, though painful, was a breakthrough. Damian began to see his body's signals – gut pain, sleepless nights – as messages from his younger self, still stuck in survival mode.[14]

His nervous system had been primed for battle since those early days of torment, colouring his adult life with hypervigilance and anxiety.

But this wasn't just a story of pathology – it was also a story of possibility. With newfound awareness, Damian began to reclaim his sense of safety. 'Between stimulus and response,' I quoted Viktor Frankl, 'there is a space. In that space lies our growth and freedom.' (see page 182) That space, long buried under automatic reactions, was now opening for him.

Through our work together, Damian learned to pause, breathe and respond deliberately rather than react automatically. Over time, he began to rewrite his narrative – shifting from constant defence to a life where he could finally feel at ease, within himself and the world around him.

Widen the gap

The 'widen the gap' exercise revolves around creating mental and emotional space between a stimulus (what happens to us) and our reaction to that stimulus. The goal is to cultivate a deliberate pause, which allows for thoughtful responses instead of automatic, habitual reactions.

- **Observe the stimulus:** Whether it's a stress trigger or a moment of joy, begin by simply observing the external event and your initial reaction. In Damian's case, this could be his work pressure or his gut pain surfacing.
- **Create a pause:** The 'gap' is the mental space where you refrain from immediately reacting. Take a moment to notice what's happening both externally (the stressful event) and internally (your physical and emotional reactions).
- **Engage mindfully:** Within this pause, consciously engage with your thoughts, feelings and bodily sensations. In the narrative, Damian begins to do this when he becomes more aware of how his gut pain and anxiety are linked to his past. This gap allows him to reflect rather than react impulsively.
- **Choose your response:** Instead of reacting in the usual way you can now choose a new, more considered response. Over time, this can break the cycle of automatic stress responses and rewire more adaptive, calm reactions.

For positive experiences, the exercise works similarly but with a focus on savouring. Instead of rushing through moments of joy, accomplishment or peace, you pause to deepen your awareness of those feelings:

- **Notice the good:** When something positive happens – whether it's as small as a warm cup of tea or as significant as a personal achievement – pause and consciously notice the emotions or sensations it evokes.

- **Stay with the feeling:** Rather than immediately moving on to the next task, allow yourself to linger with the positive emotions. Take a deep breath and notice how your body feels in this moment.
- **Amplify the positive:** Through conscious awareness, the positive experience becomes more vivid and lasting in your mind. The more you 'widen the gap' and savour positive emotions, the easier it becomes to access those feelings during difficult times, reinforcing your emotional resilience.

In Damian's case, learning to 'widen the gap' would help him shift from reacting out of habit (e.g., being constantly on edge) to responding from a place of calm and awareness. In time, he might not only manage his stress better but also find ways to truly enjoy the small victories and moments of peace in his life.

It didn't start with you

Many formative experiences occur before we can form clear memories, shaping how our bodies manage stress. During pregnancy, a mother's stress can influence her child's lifelong ability to regulate cortisol. This isn't about blaming mothers but highlights the need for stronger societal support during pregnancy, given the long-term impact.

Stress during pregnancy can elevate cortisol levels, which cross the placenta and affect the baby's developing brain, particularly areas that regulate stress. This can disrupt the development of the hypothalamic-pituitary-adrenal (HPA) axis, making the child's stress response more reactive. As they grow, they may overproduce cortisol or struggle to return to baseline after stress, leading to issues like disturbed sleep, heightened anxiety and difficulty managing everyday stressors.

No one is immune to stress or potential trauma, regardless of their social status. As Professor Robert Sapolsky poignantly points out, 'If you want to increase your chances of stress-related diseases (which I would link sleep issues with), make sure you don't inadvertently allow yourself to be born poor.'[15]

Poverty, increasingly common in today's unequal society, intensifies stress. The autonomic nervous system doesn't distinguish between privilege and deprivation – it simply perceives danger and holds on to that stress.

Childhood adversity can further sensitise the nervous system, making it more reactive to stress later in life. The Adverse Childhood Experiences (ACE) study identifies ten experiences that significantly impact long-term health outcomes, including mental health issues, heart disease and sleep disorders like insomnia[16] (see page 266 for you to work out your own ACE score), and organises them into ten questions, known as the ACE Questionnaire. Higher ACE scores are associated with a range of problems – obesity, mental health issues, heart disease, cancer and decreased immune system efficiency. They can significantly impact sleep patterns and contribute to persistent insomnia and other sleep disorders. One study published in *BMC Public Health* found that higher ACE scores were associated with a greater likelihood of persistent insomnia. It also found that supportive and nurturing environments could mitigate some of the adverse effects of ACEs on sleep.[17]

A high ACE score doesn't mean a negative outcome is inevitable, and stress from other sources can have similar effects. Chronic stress and early adversity can disrupt cortisol levels, making it harder to relax, fall asleep, stay asleep or wake feeling rested.

These stories reveal a simple truth: our days shape our nights. Safety and connection are essential for restful sleep, as mental health and the ability to regulate cortisol depend on feeling secure. Every living being seeks a safe harbour – a place where they can drop anchor and truly be present in the world. This sense of safety, cultivated through daily practices, is necessary for achieving restful sleep.

The importance of safety: Rayann's trauma

Imagine a pyramid representing your needs: at its base are essentials like food, water and shelter, but right above them is your need for safety and security (as outlined in polyvagal theory (PVT)). Psychologist Abraham Maslow developed the hierarchy of needs to explain how, just as a house needs a firm foundation, at a basic level, we all need a sense of safety and security to thrive.[18] At its core, your drive for safety and security is about survival. In more primitive times, lacking shelter and safety meant you couldn't be sure you'd live to see the next day. No wonder you still have such a strong need to feel safe and secure. If you're worried about money, where you'll sleep at night or whether your job will still be there tomorrow, the ground is shaking beneath your feet. When you feel unsafe, focusing on anything else is difficult. Your mind and body are wired to put safety first, sounding the alarm when this fundamental need is threatened. It is hard to sleep well if you feel unsafe.

Rayann grew up in a war zone, where her basic need for safety was never met. Now in her 20s, she struggles with insomnia and panic attacks, her nervous system still stuck in survival mode. Sleep, when it comes, is restless and brief, and her days are punctuated by panic attacks that strike without warning.

Most of the time, Rayann feels shut down and numb, like she's running on empty, but every now and then, she'll suddenly spike into a state of intense stress or panic. It's like her body hasn't got the message that the danger is over and keeps acting as if she's still in the middle of it.

In one of our early sessions, I asked her, 'Rayann, where do you feel safest in your home?' She looked at me with a mix of curiosity and resignation. 'I'm not sure I ever really feel safe,' she admitted. 'Even when I know I'm OK, there's this constant feeling . . . like I need to be ready to run.'

Her reaction said it all. Before we could even think about tackling her sleep issues, we had to address that constant sense of unease and help her body feel safe again. We started small, using grounding techniques – simple things to bring her back to the present. I suggested she try holding a piece of ice, running her fingers over a soft fabric or pressing her feet firmly into the floor.

These little steps were more powerful than they seemed, gently reminding her nervous system that the danger she'd once faced wasn't here anymore.

Interrupt the stress response:

Doing something physical like holding ice or feeling a soft fabric works because it taps into your sense of touch, giving your brain something real and immediate to focus on. It's a way to shift attention away from overwhelming thoughts about the past or future and bring you back to what's happening right now.

Send safety signals to the brain:

Pressing your feet firmly into the floor or engaging with textures sends signals to the brain through the somatosensory system, reinforcing a sense of physical stability and safety. This can help the nervous system 'realise' that there's no immediate danger.

But grounding exercises were only the beginning. 'Let's talk about your space,' I suggested. 'Could you bring in some pictures of your bedroom and living area? Maybe we can find ways to make it feel more secure, more like a refuge.'

She laughed a little wryly. 'Who knew better sleep might mean re-designing my room?'

In our next session, Rayann brought the photos. We talked about the small changes that could make a big difference – adding a weighted blanket for its comforting pressure, maybe an indoor fountain for its soothing sound. 'What about the lighting?' I asked. 'Warmer bulbs might make the space feel more inviting, less harsh.'

We also discussed practical measures like adding locks or rearranging furniture to create clear, accessible exit paths. For Rayann, knowing how to escape – even if it wasn't necessary – gave her a much-needed sense of control. 'It's not about expecting danger,' I told her, 'but about knowing you're prepared, just in case.'

Then there was the TV. 'I can't sleep without it on,' she confessed. 'It's like . . . I need the noise, the sense that someone's there.'

'That makes sense. The TV isn't just background noise – it's company. What if you tried setting a timer so it turns off after you fall asleep? We can work on lowering the volume gradually, too.'

These adjustments weren't just about aesthetics or habits but about creating an environment that told Rayann's nervous system, 'You are safe here.' As we made these changes, she noticed a shift. Sleep came a little easier, panic attacks became less frequent, and for the first time in years, she started to feel a glimmer of calm.

Our work together was about much more than just redesigning a room. It was about giving Rayann the tools to reshape her internal landscape and help her feel safe in her own skin and home. 'This is just the beginning,' I reminded her. 'But it's a big step. When you finally feel safe, your body and mind will start to settle.'

Like those of Damian, Perry and Clary, Rayann's journey highlights a simple but profound truth: healing begins with safety. When we create a space – both physically and emotionally – where we feel secure, our nervous systems can finally relax, sleep improves and true recovery can begin.

What wires together, fires together

Fundamental to my work is my knowing that the brain and body are constantly changing; we are not fixed entities. Without that understanding, I couldn't do what I do. Repeated activation of neural pathways strengthens them, forming new connections and habits. Yes, it can take time – but thanks to neuroplasticity, your brain is changeable because, according to Hebb's Rule, 'cells that fire together wire together.'[19] This principle has become a cornerstone of neuroscience, explaining how our brains adapt and rewire through experience.

Imagine a neural pathway – a thought pattern – as an ancient stream. We begin by placing a rock in the stream to change its course. Initially, one rock doesn't make much difference, but over time, as more rocks are added, the stream's path is gradually redirected. This illustrates neuroplasticity: small, consistent changes lead to significant transformations.

Build positive neural pathways in 5,4,3,2,1

This simple mindfulness exercise helps you connect with the present moment by engaging all five senses. Take a moment to sit or lie quietly somewhere you can't be disturbed.

- **5** things you can see. Look around and name five things you can see. Focus on their colours, shapes or textures.
- **4** things you can touch. Notice four things you can feel. It could be the texture of your clothes, the warmth of a mug or the surface of a table.
- **3** things you can hear. Listen for three distinct sounds around you, like the hum of an appliance, birds chirping or distant traffic.
- **2** things you can smell. Identify two scents. If you can't smell anything at the moment, take a deep breath or recall a favourite smell.
- **1** thing you can taste. Focus on one thing you can taste. Take a sip of water, chew gum or simply notice the lingering taste of toothpaste in your mouth.

Resist the urge to rush. Focus on each sensation as you experience it. This exercise grounds you in the here and now, calming your mind and reducing stress. It's a powerful but simple tool to build resilience and bring moments of peace into your day.

The dreaded 3–5 a.m. waking

There are *so* many reasons that you are awake: stress, depression, hyperarousal, hormones, hunger, food timing, alcohol, sleep apnea, noise, thirst, acid reflux, peri-menopause and menopause, prostate, irregular sleep patterns . . . the list goes on. Brief wake-ups during sleep cycles are actually normal, but they become problematic when they stretch out and your mind starts racing. Understanding why this happens – and how to manage it – is key to reclaiming restful sleep. When I take workshops and ask people if they find themselves awake around 3 a.m., most hands go up – and most people are surprised but relieved to see that it is common.

That's not to say it makes it OK, and how each of us respond to it varies greatly. Sleep is the tale of two halves. At this point of the night most people are transitioning from the first half of the night where you get the most deep sleep into the second half with lighter REM sleep. At this time, cortisol – your body's primary stress hormone – naturally begins to rise, while melatonin, the hormone that promotes sleep, starts to decline. The 'sleep pressure' that built up over the day (caused by the accumulation of adenosine in the brain) is also wearing off. Under normal conditions, this gentle rise in cortisol helps prepare your body to wake up in the morning. But if you're already stressed, that extra cortisol can push you into full wakefulness earlier than needed.

Ideally, you will wake up, notice you are awake, groggily stumble to the bathroom then back to bed to drop off again. It may be that you are a bit more awake than that so the falling asleep again takes a bit longer, but it happens. Worst-case scenario is that you wake up with a start, heart racing, and the panic begins. There are multiple levels of what happens to people.

One explanation for how we respond to this waking is the 'Mind After Midnight' hypothesis.[20] It suggests that during the early hours of the morning, our cognitive and emotional states are more negatively skewed, making us more prone to worry and anxiety.[21] So, when you wake up at 3 a.m., your brain may be more likely to fixate on concerns or stressors, which can quickly spiral into full-blown stress, making it harder to fall back asleep.

The more stressed you feel about being awake, the higher your cortisol levels rise, making it even harder to drift back to sleep. And the stress from a poor night's sleep often carries over into the next day, increasing the chances of waking up again at the same time the following night.

Other reasons why it might happen

During the night, blood sugar naturally drops, but if it dips too low, it can trigger the release of cortisol and adrenaline, potentially waking you up. This is more common in people with irregular eating patterns or restrictive diets. If you often wake around 3 a.m., a small, balanced bedtime snack – such as whole-grain toast with almond butter – may help stabilise blood sugar levels overnight. However, it's important to assess whether hunger is the cause, as waking at this time can stem from other factors, like stress or disrupted circadian rhythms. If needed, consulting a nutrition professional for tailored advice can be helpful.

Alcohol is a common sleep disruptor, especially if consumed close to bedtime. While it may initially help you fall asleep, it interferes with sleep quality and can cause early morning wake-ups as your body metabolises it. Alcohol disrupts REM sleep and can lead to more fragmented sleep, which is why many people find themselves wide awake around 3 a.m. after an evening drink.

Hormonal shifts, such as those related to menopause, perimenopause or adrenal issues, can make you more prone to early morning awakenings. During menopause, for example, hot flushes and night sweats can occur in the early morning hours, causing disrupted sleep. If this is a regular issue, consult with your healthcare provider for advice on managing these hormonal changes.

I know I keep going on about it, but a consistent sleep routine is essential. If you continue to struggle with early morning wake-ups, consider sleep restriction (see page 19). This technique involves limiting your time in bed to consolidate sleep, which can help improve sleep efficiency over time. If these wake-ups persist, it might be worth considering whether underlying issues, like sleep apnea or hormonal imbalances (the menopause is notorious for wrecking sleep at 3 a.m.), could be contributing. A visit to your GP can help rule out these factors.

Waking up at 3 a.m. doesn't have to be a nightly ordeal or become a brutally early start to your day. By understanding the reasons behind these wake-ups and practising effective strategies, you can break the cycle of stress and sleep loss. It might be that it's part of your normal sleep pattern. It's about creating a sense of safety and having a plan in place to guide you back to sleep or to handle wakefulness if and when you do wake up.

What you seek to avoid grows stronger

Sleep deprivation can feel deeply isolating, especially when it robs you of REM sleep – the kind that helps process emotions and maintain

Getting back to sleep

The key to breaking this cycle is preparation and practice – especially during the waking hours. There is nothing worse than trying to implement a coping strategy when you are stressed at 3 a.m.:

- **Physical grounding:** Focus on your body – feel the texture of your sheets or the coolness of your pillow. This can anchor you in the present moment and ease racing thoughts.
- **Mental grounding:** Distract your mind with simple cognitive tasks like counting backwards from 100 or naming objects around the room, or do the 5,4,3,2,1 exercise on page 173. This helps shift your focus away from anxious thoughts.
- **Safe-place visualisation:** Imagine a place where you feel completely safe and secure. Visualise this space to calm your mind and body.
- **Positive imagery:** Focus on positive thoughts or outcomes. This can help counteract the negative bias of waking at this time.
- **Breathing exercises:** Practise deep, slow breathing to activate your parasympathetic nervous system and lower cortisol levels, helping you relax back into sleep.
- **Listen to yoga nidra or progressive relaxation:** These guided meditations can deeply relax your body and mind, making it easier to drift back to sleep (see pages 272–5).
- **Get out of bed:** Go and do something you enjoy until your next sleep window comes along and you feel sleepy again.

Worst-case scenario – you can't get back to sleep. OK, this isn't ideal but there are some plus points. Remember, the longer you are awake, the more sleep pressure builds up and the following night you should get a recovery sleep. You might want to go to bed a little earlier – don't go to bed hugely earlier as that's not a solution.

Be mindful that it's not a licence to start work. That will raise your stress levels and start to create a tricky cycle.

Take care of yourself during the day and take a nap if you need to (and aren't doing sleep restriction).

Strategies to help with the 3 a.m. wake-up

- At 3 a.m., your mind can magnify worries, making them feel urgent and overwhelming. But remember, a thought is just a thought. It doesn't mean it's real, especially in the quiet of night. What seems critical now often feels minor in the light of day.
- Remember, your mind is vulnerable at this hour, prone to drifting into anxious places. Think of your thoughts as clouds – just let them drift by without chasing after them. This simple acknowledgement can help you find calm and settle back into rest.
- Waking at this time may feel isolating, but it's important to remember that you're not alone. Many people wake up around 3 a.m.; it's a normal part of the sleep cycle. I know you might feel like you're the only one awake but countless others are experiencing the same moment of wakefulness.
- If you're making changes to your sleep routine or coming off sleep medication, you might experience rebound insomnia, where old sleep issues resurface temporarily. Have soothing strategies ready, like breathing exercises or grounding techniques, to ease you through these nights.
- Waking at 3 a.m. can feel isolating, but instead of resisting it, can you embrace the quiet? The stillness of the night can offer a moment of reflection or even gratitude. Can you be curious about this solitude, to see what else you might experience?
- If you're still awake after 20 minutes, leave the bed. Do a calming activity – like reading or listening to soft music – then return when you feel sleepy. This helps your brain break the association between bed and restlessness.

Remember, the thoughts can feel super-real, but they might just be passing visitors. Let them come and go, and trust that sleep will find its way back to you.

healthy social connections. Without it, you might find yourself stuck in negative thoughts, misreading interactions and withdrawing from others. This withdrawal can increase loneliness, creating a painful cycle where poor sleep feeds isolation, and isolation worsens sleep.

Loneliness can also blur the boundaries of your day. Without the energy or motivation to engage with the world, you might stay up late scrolling on your phone or watching TV to escape your thoughts, or nap during the day to ease sadness or exhaustion. These habits, while understandable, can confuse your body's internal clock and make restful sleep even harder to achieve. Over time, the quiet hours of the night can feel endless, amplifying the sense of being alone.

At 3 a.m., when the world feels still and you feel most vulnerable, it's natural to reach for small comforts – social media, snacks or TV. These offer temporary relief, but they can make things harder. Social media may heighten feelings of inadequacy, screen light disrupts your sleep further, and substances like alcohol or nicotine can destabilise your sleep cycle.

Avoiding the stress or worry that wakes you often reinforces its hold on you. It teaches your brain to associate wakefulness with tension, increasing the likelihood of future 3 a.m. wake-ups. Similarly, distractions like overworking or procrastinating during the day can spill over into the night, keeping your mind restless when you need peace the most.

Breaking this cycle requires compassion for yourself. It's not about forcing sleep or pushing away discomfort – it's about gently acknowledging what's weighing on you. You don't need to have all the answers in the moment, but by being present with your feelings instead of avoiding them, you can slowly build resilience and restore balance. Facing discomfort with kindness creates space for healing, helping both your days and nights feel lighter.

Feel the fear and do it anyway

Remember, the more you avoid something, the stronger its hold on you becomes. Coping mechanisms like excessive screen time, substance use or even avoiding social interactions might offer quick relief, but they often exacerbate the underlying issues. Facing your discomfort, especially at 3 a.m. when the world feels quiet and lonely, is essential to breaking the cycle of stress and sleep disruption.

As Susan Jeffers suggests in her book *Feel the Fear and Do It Anyway*,[22] embracing discomfort is a natural part of growth. By facing your 3 a.m. wake-ups head-on, without resorting to avoidance, you not only improve your sleep but also build resilience and confidence in your ability to handle stress. Over time, these efforts will transform those lonely, anxious hours into moments of quiet reflection and eventual rest.

One truth stands out at the heart of this journey: managing stress is essential for restful sleep. Whether it's Damian's hypervigilance, Perry's anger, Clary's exhaustion or Rayann's trauma, the common thread is the universal need for safety, connection and regulation. Each of them seeks a sense of grounding – a place of calm where sleep, and ultimately peace, can be found. Their stories remind us that we all need to feel safe enough to let go, rest and heal.

Reimagining rest and recuperation

When was the last time you felt truly rested? Not just caught up on sleep, but genuinely refreshed? It's a harsh realisation, isn't it? We've been operating under a flawed model for too long. The old notion says, 'work hard, then recover by playing hard.' But real wellbeing isn't about oscillating between extremes. It's about nurturing a daily rhythm of rest, play and meaningful engagement, so you never reach the brink of burnout.

We think we understand rest and recuperation (R&R) – a whole night's sleep, a weekend off, maybe a holiday. But R&R is about more than the hours your eyes are closed. It's about how you spend your waking hours. Are you allowing yourself moments to pause and reset throughout the day, or are you simply pushing until you collapse into bed, hoping sleep will save you?

Most people think being 'awake' means simply not being asleep. But are you truly awake? Are you engaged with life, mentally alert and emotionally OK? Or are you scraping through tasks, wringing yourself dry of energy, waiting for sleep to fix it all? If you're collapsing into bed, you're not set up to recover through sleep – you're charged up with cortisol, stuck in survival mode.

As children, summers felt endless. But as we grow older, time seems to shrink, becoming a limited resource. We spend our waking hours juggling work, personal obligations and the quest for meaningful experiences, often at the cost of rest and relaxation. This sense of 'time poverty' leaves many of us feeling constantly rushed and underslept.[23] I've emphasised the importance of rest throughout this book, but did you know it can take many forms?

The seven types of rest

When you feel exhausted or wrung out, your first thought is often, 'I just need more sleep.' But while sleep is vital, it's not always the complete answer. Sometimes what you truly need isn't more sleep but a different type of restoration. Dr Saundra Dalton-Smith, physician and author, identifies seven distinct types of rest to fully restore our mind, body and soul.[24]

1. **Physical rest:** Your body needs a break. This might take the form of a good nap or a long night's sleep, but it could also be something simple like stretching, doing yoga or just sitting down for a moment and letting yourself breathe.
2. **Mental rest:** Is your mind always racing? You need mental rest. Take a break from overthinking – step away from the to-do list, let yourself zone out or just give your brain a chance to slow down and reset.
3. **Sensory rest:** Screens, noise, bright lights – it's a lot, isn't it? Turn off the notifications, dim the lights or grab some earplugs. Give your senses a little peace and quiet.
4. **Creative rest:** When was the last time you felt inspired? Creative rest comes from reconnecting with things that spark joy – art, nature, music or anything new and exciting that reminds you of the beauty in the world.
5. **Emotional rest:** You carry so much, don't you? Emotional rest might be about letting go of the pressure to keep everyone else happy or creating space to feel your feelings without judgement.

6. **Social rest:** Not all relationships fill you up. Social rest is about spending time with the people who make you feel good and setting boundaries with those who don't.

7. **Spiritual rest:** This is where you find your deeper sense of meaning. Maybe it's faith, meditation or just taking a moment to feel like you're part of something bigger than yourself..

I always ask people what they do for rest, and it's a stark truth that very few can tell me. Often, the answer is that 'I haven't got time.' Sometimes, just knowing that rest isn't limited to sleep can open the door to feeling more balanced and refreshed. Our approach to rest is as broken as the grind we're trying to escape from. We treat it like an emergency brake, slamming it on when we're already crashing. If you don't slam it on yourself, your body will do it for you – think of the illness that suddenly hits the moment you start your holiday. But what if rest weren't just an antidote to exhaustion? What if it were something you cultivated every day, a rhythm that fuels you rather than a response to depletion?

Let's have some fun

Fun isn't just for weekends or kids – it's your brain's ultimate reset button. When you laugh, play or let go, your body shifts from 'fight-or-flight' to 'rest-and-digest'. It's not indulgence; it's survival in disguise. Science agrees, but you don't need studies to tell you how good a belly laugh feels.

Even in tough times, humour sneaks in, offering relief. A dark joke in a dire moment isn't just funny; it's a lifeline reminding you that you're human, resilient and here. And when you laugh, even cynically, you tell your body, 'It's OK to relax.'

Fun doesn't happen on a schedule – you can't calendar joy for 3 p.m. or force a chuckle at 3 a.m. But it thrives when you loosen your grip. Watch a silly video, say yes to something spontaneous or dive into a playful hobby. Fun doesn't need permission; it just needs space.

When I bring this up with clients, there's often resistance. Fun can't be forced, right? You can't schedule joy like a meeting.

As kids, we could shift from tears to laughter in a heartbeat, but what happened? As adults, where does that ability go?

Fun thrives in the spaces where expectations loosen. But fun can slip through the cracks if you don't make room for it.

The secret lies in loosening your grip. Fun doesn't come from control – it comes from letting go. Maybe it's pretending for a moment to see what happens, trying a hobby or saying yes to a spontaneous invitation. These are the spaces where fun surprises you.

Think back to when you were completely absorbed in something that made you laugh and feel alive. It wasn't just a fleeting feel-good moment – it was your body resetting itself. You were pulling yourself out of 'fight-or-flight' mode and into genuine recovery.

It's easy to forget about fun as life becomes more serious – more responsibilities, pressures and to-dos on your list. And yet, the irony is that fun is as essential to your wellbeing as sleep and nutrition. Research from Yamagata University in Japan found that people who laugh less than once a month have nearly double the risk of dying compared with those who laugh at least once a week.[25] Laughter, play and joy are built into your neurochemistry. They're not optional, they're essential.

You might be thinking, 'I don't have time for fun – I'm too busy,' or perhaps life feels too overwhelming and the idea of play touches a nerve. Yet, the importance of play, fun and humour is widely recognised across various fields – even in the most trying times. Holocaust survivor and psychiatrist Viktor Frankl spoke of humour as a tool for survival, while Brené Brown emphasises joy as a cornerstone of resilience.

Fun is a tool for deep recovery. It's not just for kids or weekends – it's for everyone, every day, especially for those struggling to sleep. Play rewires your brain to relax and recover. When you allow yourself moments of joy, you signal to your nervous system that it's OK to let go. You're giving your body permission to release the day's tension, setting yourself up for the kind of sleep that genuinely restores.

So, here's the paradox: the better you are at being awake – fully engaged, alive and joyful – the easier it will be to sleep at night. Rest and play aren't distractions from life; they are how you prepare your mind and body to shut down when it's time. It's permission to cultivate a life that feels like your own again.

Summary

It's natural to question whether the subtle strategies I suggest can make a meaningful difference. You might wonder: Can small shifts in routine really help with sleep disturbances, anxiety or even depression? Shouldn't the solution be more robust, perhaps involving medication?

These doubts are valid. But I assure you, small, consistent changes – grounded in both research and experience – can have a profound impact over time. It may seem modest, but practising these strategies regularly can transform how you sleep, feel and manage the pressures of daily life. Sometimes, the most potent changes begin with the simplest actions.

Many believe that a pill is the ultimate solution to their problems, and practices like breathwork or mindfulness can seem insufficient. This scepticism is understandable in a culture that values resilience and constant productivity over restoration and wellbeing. In the midst of suffering, everything feels overwhelming, and it's tempting to search for a doctor or medication to 'fix' things. However, this belief that medicine holds all the answers is flawed.

Sleep issues often leave you feeling powerless, especially after years of trying to fix the problem with little success. It's easy to arrive with a mindset of helplessness, yearning to be fixed. Anxiety, burnout and depression are rampant in our modern world. We compare ourselves with others – co-workers who seem alert and efficient, parents at the school gate who appear to have everything under control. But as someone who sees behind the curtain of people's lives, I know those calm exteriors can mask inner chaos.

Take it bit by bit, focus on what you can during the day so that sleep takes care of itself.

Actionable steps

- Create a consistent morning routine to help reduce stress and wake up smoothly.
- Spend time each day doing mindfulness exercises and talking positively to yourself.
- Use a journal or app to track your feelings about stress and sleep, and find ways to think more positively.
- Use techniques like focusing on your senses to help you stay present and calm.
- Ensure your living space feels safe and cosy to help reduce anxiety.
- Build and maintain meaningful relationships with family and friends.
- Daily glimmers: reflect on and write about three positive moments each day.
- Slowly confront things that stress you out to build resilience and avoid avoidance habits.
- Do activities that make you feel good and help rewire your brain for positivity.
- Establish a consistent and calming morning routine to regulate cortisol levels and reduce stress.
- Plan for what you will do when you are awake in the night to feel in control.

CHAPTER SIX

The sensory pathway to sound sleep

Humans are fundamentally sensory creatures. Our emotions and senses respond to and shape daily experiences, and how you feel about them can significantly impact your sleep. While we commonly recognise five or six senses – sight, smell, taste, touch, sound and the sixth, proprioception, meaning an awareness of the body in space – eco-psychologist Michael J. Cohen suggests there may be as many as 53.[1] The senses are our primary way of interacting with and interpreting the world.

Think about the sense of smell; it can evoke powerful memories and emotions. The aroma of a specific flower might transport you back to your grandparents' home, filling you with warmth and nostalgia. Similarly, the sound of a loved one's voice can provide comfort and security, instantly calming you in moments of stress.

In today's world, where many of us spend most of the time indoors (people in North America and Europe spend about 90 per cent of their time indoors; in countries like the UAE, this can rise to nearly 100 per cent during certain seasons[2]), our senses can suffer from a lack of natural stimulation. This imbalance can make your senses either overly sensitive or under-stimulated. Sensory overload and desensitisation can be closely linked to anxiety and depression. When your senses are overstimulated, it can lead to a constant state of heightened alertness, which fuels anxiety and makes it difficult to relax. On the other hand, desensitisation, where you become numb or detached from your surroundings, can feed into feelings of depression and disconnection.

Both states – overload and numbness – can disrupt emotional balance. Sensory overload may keep you in fight-or-flight mode, draining energy and making it hard to wind down, while desensitisation can leave you feeling flat and disengaged, making it challenging to find joy in daily life. When things become unbalanced, it may seem easier to avoid human contact and live life in the digital realm. However, by avoiding physical interaction, you lose something profound. Without human touch and face-to-face communication, you become disconnected from your inner self, making it harder to connect emotionally and maintain mental wellbeing.

You can help calm yourself by paying attention to what your body feels, your breathing and how you move.

Our brains are constantly picking up clues from our surroundings and using them to predict what's coming next. This means you can lower stress and sleep better by adjusting the sensory environment around you – not just at night, but all day. Small changes, like soft lighting, gentle sounds or calming scents, can help guide your brain towards relaxation and rest instead of keeping it on high alert.

Don't think – feel

Think about the soothing sound of ocean waves or the gentle touch of a loved one's hand – these sensory moments can make you feel calm and comforted. This phenomenon, known as the 'felt sense', is about tuning in to your body's physical sensations and understanding their connection to your emotional states. It's a practice of presence, an invitation to engage fully with the here and now, allowing your body to guide you to a place of peace.

Our sensory environment profoundly impacts our emotional and cognitive states. Natural settings like green spaces or bodies of water can significantly reduce stress and promote relaxation, while harsh sounds might cause tension and agitation. Research shows that viewing water, even for a short period, can lower blood pressure and heart rate, enhancing relaxation. This state, referred to as 'Blue Mind' by marine biologist Dr Wallace Nichols, underscores our deep, intrinsic connection to water.[3] The sight and sound of water can trigger a positive brain response, promoting rest and relaxation.

Dr Shige Oishi's research suggests that different personality types may gravitate towards different natural settings – extroverts often find solace in the expansive energy of the beach. At the same time, introverts may seek the solitude and serenity of the mountains.[4]

Blue Mind relaxation ritual for better sleep

Allow 15–20 minutes.

You can do this at any time of the day or night. If possible, have a photo of mountains, the ocean or any place that you have a positive association with, or play a recording of gentle ocean sounds.

1. Close your eyes and take slow, deep breaths. Inhale through your nose for a count of four, hold for a count of four, and exhale through your mouth for a count of six.
2. Repeat this breathing pattern for a few minutes, allowing your body and mind to relax.
3. With your eyes closed, visualise a perfect day by the sea. Picture the gentle waves lapping against the shore, the cool breeze and the smell of salt in the air.
4. Imagine yourself sitting or lying down on a soft, sandy beach. Feel the sun's warmth on your skin and your body sinking into the soft sand.
5. Focus on each of your senses one by one, imagining how they are engaged in this tranquil beach scene.
   - **Sight:** Picture the colours of the sky, the shimmering water and the distant horizon.
   - **Sound:** Listen to the rhythmic sound of the waves, the calls of seagulls and the gentle rustling of palm leaves.
   - **Touch:** Feel the soft sand beneath you, the cool water touching your feet and the gentle breeze on your skin.
   - **Smell:** Breathe in the fresh, salty air mixed with the faint scent of tropical flowers.
   - **Taste:** Imagine tasting a hint of salt in the air, perhaps paired with a cool, refreshing drink.

As you focus on each sense, allow yourself to sink deeper into relaxation, feeling more and more at peace. You may have fallen asleep by now, but if not, gradually bring your visualisation to a close, maintaining the sense of calm and relaxation you've created. Take a few deep breaths, slowly and deeply.

- Repeat this ritual nightly to create a consistent, calming bedtime routine.
- If you have trouble visualising, simply focus on the sound of the ocean or even your own breathing.
- Use soft, calming background sounds like ocean waves or gentle music to enhance the experience.

Sensory overload

'Everything is too much,' Jenna said, stepping into my office, her words spilling out in a rush. 'The honking cars, the flickering lights, the endless chatter at work. Even the smell of people's perfume on the bus. By the time I get home, it's all still there – like a buzzsaw reverberating round my head. When my head hits the pillow, I can still hear those voices, still feel the vibrations. I know it's not real, but it's got into my bones. Even though I know they aren't there, I can still smell the smells.'

Autistic individuals, like Jenna, often have a heightened sensory sensitivity, making the world feel overwhelmingly intense. This predisposes them to insomnia, as sensory overload can activate the autonomic nervous system (ANS), keeping the body in a fight-or-flight state that disrupts relaxation and sleep. Co-occurring conditions like generalised anxiety disorder (GAD), PTSD, and ADHD further compound hyperarousal, making restful sleep even harder to achieve.

Research suggests that some autistic individuals may have irregular circadian rhythms or lower melatonin levels, complicating the sleep–wake cycle and making it harder for them to fall asleep or wake up refreshed. Sleep deprivation worsens sensory sensitivities, turning manageable stimuli into overwhelming challenges.

Paradoxically, people with autism can find night-time to be a refuge, free from social and sensory demands. However, this sense of safety can lead to a reluctance to sleep, as the quiet hours offer rare peace. Studies reveal that up to 80 per cent of autistic children and 50–70 per cent of autistic adults experience significant sleep issues, such as insomnia, disrupted sleep or irregular patterns, highlighting the pervasive impact of autism on rest.[5]

I listened as Jenna described a world that felt as if it were closing in on her, and told her that I thought she was experiencing sensory overload. 'When our brains are bombarded with too much input – too many sights, sounds, smells – it can feel as if we're under attack,' I told her. 'The brain reacts by triggering the fight, flight or freeze response. It's no wonder you feel unsafe, fearful, panicky. And when night falls, the echoes of the day linger, making it almost impossible to find rest.'

I asked if there were any specific triggers that made the overload feel worse.

'Crowded places,' she replied without hesitation. 'Even just going to the supermarket leaves me feeling frazzled. Bright lights, loud noises, and when I try to read or listen to something at the same time, it's overwhelming. My skin feels tight, prickly – I can't stand it.'

I could sense how deeply she was affected. Anxiety often manifests physically. It's not just the mind that suffers; the body takes the hit, too. Sensory overload can feel like an internal storm – skin that once felt neutral now prickles with discomfort, and nerves that were once quiet now scream with irritation. The ANS, already on high alert, amplifies every sensation. And then there's the sleep deprivation, which only makes the storm worse, distorting how sensory information is processed and turning minor irritations into overwhelming onslaughts.

Jenna also has a PTSD diagnosis, for which she has been undergoing eye movement desensitisation and reprocessing (EMDR),[6] as well as generalised anxiety disorder. We've been exploring different coping strategies and reframing techniques, including this exercise, which I call 'talk to the hand'.

Talk to the hand

- **Focus on your hand:** hold up one of your hands in front of your face, allowing your arm to rest comfortably. If that feels odd or if it isn't something you can do in the present moment, just place your hand where you can see it. Look at your hand as if seeing it for the first time, noticing its shape, colour and unique features.
- **Observe the details:** notice the lines on your palm, the texture of your skin, the way light reflects off your nails and the subtle movements your hand might make without you even realising.
- **Feel the sensations:** close your eyes and shift your focus from visual observation to sensation. Feel any tingling, warmth or pulsing in your hand. Pay attention to the feelings that arise, observing them without judgement.
- **Connect with the rhythms:** as you concentrate on your hand, try to synchronise your breathing with any rhythmic sensations you feel, like the pulse in your fingertips. Inhale deeply and imagine the breath flowing to your hand, exhaling slowly and feeling a sense of relaxation spreading from your hand to the rest of your body.

Jenna really connected with this exercise, commenting on how she immediately saw that she could use it as a distraction in the supermarket. She also noticed how it eases the feeling of tightness in her skin – she can see her skin, and she knows it is OK.

People with conditions like sensory processing disorder, generalised anxiety disorder, ADHD, autism or PTSD are more prone to sensory overload. Anxiety and sensory overload often fuel each other, creating a cycle that's hard to break. When you're anxious, your senses are already heightened, making overload more likely. In turn, sensory overload can trigger or worsen anxiety, creating a feedback loop. Understanding how these two are linked is crucial for managing both. By using calming techniques or making your environment more sensory-friendly, you can help reduce this pressure and find relief.

You're probably familiar with how sensory overload looks in children – meltdowns, tantrums, crying and screaming, often mistaken for misbehaviour. But what about adults? We may not throw ourselves on the floor like a two-year-old, but we still have our own versions of tantrums, even if they look quite different. What do adult 'tantrums' really look like?

Instead of a full-blown meltdown, you might find yourself experiencing sudden mood swings or reacting far more strongly to minor annoyances than seems reasonable. Ever snapped at someone over something trivial or felt overwhelming frustration at a small inconvenience? That's your body and mind being pushed past their capacity to cope – essentially, your adult version of a tantrum.

You might notice a growing sense of anxiety, restlessness or nervous energy that makes it hard to relax or focus. Sometimes, it's not about snapping but feeling like you need to withdraw or escape – maybe shutting yourself off from others, avoiding conversations or just wanting to be left alone. Your 'tantrum' could look like leaving a gathering abruptly or scrolling endlessly through your phone to avoid engaging.

There are also physical signs. Sensory overload can show up as headaches, muscle tension, fatigue or even nausea, as your body reacts to the overload. That overwhelming sensation of being 'done' with everything? It's your system telling you it's had too much input and needs relief.

So, while you may not stomp your feet and scream, your adult tantrums may be more subtle, but no less real. Whether through irritability, withdrawal or physical discomfort, your body is signalling that you're at your limit. It's hardly surprising that enduring these symptoms will have an impact on your sleep.

Are you living in a state of overwhelm?

Step 1: Spot the overloads
Identify the sensory inputs, situations or environments that overwhelm you. Think loud noises, crowded places, bright lights – anything that makes you feel like you're in a pinball machine.

Step 2: Describe the impact

For each overload, briefly describe how it affects you. Be specific about what you notice and how it makes you feel.

Step 3: Reflect

Consider how these inputs impact your wellbeing. Note how they affect your mood, energy and focus.

Step 4: Make a plan

Create a simple plan to reduce or manage these inputs. Take breaks from noisy spots, use noise-cancelling headphones, find quieter spaces or adjust lighting. Think – 'How can I support myself?'

Step 5: Act and observe

Put your plan into action. Observe any changes in your environment and your reactions. Note improvements or challenges.

Step 6: Tweak as needed

Regularly review and adjust your plan. Fine-tune what works and discard what doesn't.

By becoming aware of what overwhelms you, you take the first step in controlling your surroundings. This awareness helps you create a more peaceful environment, making your day smoother and more focused.

Breaking down the senses

Sight

From the moment you open your eyes in the morning, the visual system kicks into high gear. Vision is the brain's most energy-intensive sense. Every glance, flicker of light or moment in front of a screen requires significant mental power. The way the news is presented today is just a small example of this becoming problematic: there is a main image, audio, a scrolling ticker of information and often another inset video – all forcing your brain to juggle multiple streams of input at once. Over time, this relentless flood of visual data places a heavy metabolic load on your brain, often leaving you overwhelmed without even realising it.

Consider how your eyes navigate busy environments, like an open-plan office or a crowded street, constantly absorbing visual stimuli like advertising, signage, people, cars and so much more. Open-plan offices aim to encourage collaboration but often lead to sensory overload. Constant visual and auditory stimuli – like conversations, movements and notifications – keep your brain in overdrive, causing mental fatigue and increased stress. The stress from processing all these details builds up quickly, leaving your brain overstimulated. If you are already stressed, your sensitivity to your surroundings increases, amplifying the visual chaos and amping up the stress response, which in turn disrupts sleep.

Remember, sensory overload leads to stress, which affects your sleep ability. You might even notice that after a day of heavy screen time, you feel more wired and have a harder time winding down before bed. Ignoring these signals – telling yourself to push through even when your focus slips and exhaustion builds – keeps your brain in overdrive, making it difficult to relax or sleep well at night.

However, there's a solution. Closing your eyes for just a few seconds or stepping away from visual stimulation throughout the day allows your brain to recover, reducing the stress buildup that contributes to poor sleep. These short breaks allow the visual cortex to reset, reducing mental fatigue and helping to prevent the cognitive overload that can spill over into sleepless nights.

The 20-20-20 Rule:

Every 20 minutes, take a 20-second break to look at something 20 feet away. It not only relaxes your eye muscles but also prevents stress from accumulating, helping to reduce tension that can interfere with sleep later.

Sound

Hearing is a powerful sense that can evoke strong emotions and explicit memories. Certain sounds can transport us back to forgotten memories, stir intense emotions and even help us feel safe while asleep. You know how sometimes you can sleep right through the hum of a fan but wake up instantly if your phone goes off or you hear a baby cry? That's because, even while we're sleeping, the brain continues to operate, filtering sounds and staying alert for anything that might mean danger.[7]

But not all sounds are so easy to ignore. If we aren't used to them, certain noises – like traffic, distant conversations, or even random creaks and clicks – can prevent us from drifting off altogether or cause brief wake-ups or changes in sleep stages.[8] Equally, if you are used to the low hum of city life, the quiet of the countryside can be unnerving. Some sounds, like soft music or a humming heater, can help us relax.[9] These comforting sounds create a bit of an auditory cocoon, blocking out sudden disruptions and making it easier to unwind.

Of course, finding this kind of peace isn't always possible, especially in shared spaces like open-plan offices or on public transport. These places can be sensory overload zones, especially if you're sensitive to noise. Picture a typical open office: phones ringing, people chatting, keyboards clacking. And then there's the latest invasion – the habit of playing TikTok videos, blasting music or taking calls on speakerphone in public spaces without headphones. It's become all too common, and in a quiet setting like an office or a train, it can feel maddeningly intrusive.

For people with heightened sensitivity to sound, like those with misophonia (a condition that causes strong emotional reactions to specific sounds, which can become a source of stress) or other sensory processing challenges, this unpredictable barrage of noise is more than just annoying; it's exhausting. The mental energy it takes to tune out or ignore these sounds can drain you and increase stress levels. I think that's why, if you're bothered by noise, investing in a good pair of noise-cancelling headphones or decent ear plugs (I always recommend the soft mouldable wax ear plugs to clients) can feel like a lifeline. If you're dealing with loud offices or crowded trains, a solid set of headphones can be one of the best investments you'll make.

Different noises

White noise spans all audible frequencies evenly, providing a consistent, static-like sound that can mask other noises across the entire sound spectrum.

> **Pink noise** has equal energy per octave, which means it emphasises lower frequencies more than higher ones, creating a sound that resembles a gentle waterfall or rain.
> **Brown noise,** or red noise, has a deeper and more robust sound, similar to the rumble of distant thunder or a strong wind.

Having a personal, almost idiosyncratic reaction to sound isn't uncommon. Each of us responds to sound differently. Some people swear by white noise to help them focus or sleep, while others can't stand it. I am often asked whether to use white (or pink or brown) noise to ease stress and block exterior sound. Recent research is polarised as, like most things, human preferences vary. It is increasingly popular, with streaming services cashing in on the trend. Still, Professor Colin Espie at the University of Oxford highlights a potential issue with continuous noise. In a newspaper interview, he commented, 'White noise is just like any other monotonous stimulation, which has been tried many times in many ways over decades, and the evidence [for its efficacy] is poor.'[10] But some swear by it, and those who hate it find they really hate it! Perhaps this polarisation is linked to the phenomenon of ASMR.

ASMR and humming

Autonomous sensory meridian response (ASMR) is a popular phenomenon that, for many, is deeply calming, but for others has the opposite effect, provoking an uncomfortable reaction. Videos may include scenarios such as watching someone stroke brushes on a microphone, folding towels or whispering – creating a unique soundscape that helps you to relax. This feeling has been described as a 'braingasm', a euphoric sensation that begins within the scalp and travels down the neck and back, like the tingling feeling of someone lightly stroking your skin. These tingles are specific to ASMR, but only around 20 per cent of people who try it will experience them. Many people find ASMR relaxing and use it to help reduce stress and anxiety or help with falling asleep. ASMR content is widely available on platforms like YouTube, where creators produce videos designed to evoke this response.

There's no one-size-fits-all answer, which makes sound so interesting – and so challenging to manage in shared spaces.

If you're wondering about options for soothing sound, you can try some simple tools beyond noise-cancelling headphones. Humming, for example, might sound too simple to be effective, but it can work wonders. When you hum, the gentle vibrations activate the parasympathetic nervous system, which is your body's built-in calming mechanism. Humming is rhythmic, grounding and has a calming quality that can help reduce anxiety. You might even want to try a quick humming meditation – just a few minutes can make a difference.

Humming meditation

Allow 5 minutes.

1. Sit or lie in a relaxed position, close your eyes and take a few deep breaths to centre yourself. You can do this on the move, shaking and swinging your body to release tension as you hum.
2. Begin to hum softly. Choose any comfortable pitch and let the humming vibration resonate throughout your body.
3. Focus on the vibration and sound, allowing them to create a sense of calm and concentration.
4. Continue humming for about five minutes. If your mind wanders, gently bring your attention to the hum and its sensations.

Tinnitus

Tinnitus is when you hear sounds like ringing, buzzing or hissing in your ears or head without any external noise to cause them. This condition can make sleeping difficult, leading to insomnia or restless nights. Stress and anxiety can make tinnitus worse, and if caused by emotional or psychological trauma, it can be particularly persistent and distressing, potentially leading to depression, anxiety and more sleep problems.[11]

Treating tinnitus usually involves managing the symptoms rather than curing the condition. Common methods include sound therapy (using background noise to drown out the tinnitus), CBT to help change how you perceive and react to the sounds, and hearing aids if you have hearing loss. Additionally, improving your sleep and managing stress can help reduce its impact.

Neurodiversity and sensory relaxation

Relaxation is as individual as a fingerprint, shaped by sensory preferences, life experiences, and even biology. While many associate calm with soft music and dim lighting, what soothes one person may overwhelm another. This diversity in relaxation strategies is strikingly illustrated in *The Accountant* (2016), where Christian Wolff, a forensic accountant who is autistic, finds calm through an intense sensory ritual involving heavy metal music, strobe lights and deep pressure.[12]

In the film, Wolff uses these tools to self-regulate after experiencing sensory overload. While this scene is dramatised for entertainment, it points to a deeper truth: relaxation is deeply personal, especially for individuals with neurodivergent sensory systems. It's worth noting, however, that Wolff's portrayal is fictional and represents just one experience on the broad and varied spectrum of autism. Understanding that sensory preferences vary widely – even within the autistic community – can help us appreciate the need for highly individualised approaches to relaxation and self-care.

For many autistic individuals, sensory experiences can feel amplified or dulled compared with neurotypical people. Some may be hyper-responsive to sensory input – startling at loud noises or feeling overwhelmed by bright lights. Others may be hypo-responsive, seeking more intense input like firm pressure or strong textures to feel grounded.

Think of it like a volume dial: for some, the sound is turned up too high, while for others, it's too low. These sensory differences aren't deficits but rather variations in how people process the world around them. For those who are hypo-responsive, activities like deep-pressure therapy or weighted blankets may help provide the sensory input they crave. For those who are hyper-responsive, quiet environments and softer stimuli may be key to finding calm.

As Chloé Hayden, the Australian author and actress, explains in a post on social media, 'The world wasn't built for me, so I built my own world.'[13] These principles tie back directly to sleep: understanding your unique sensory and emotional needs can help you create a night-time routine that feels safe, soothing and restorative, setting the stage for a more peaceful transition to sleep.

Routines and rituals are another powerful tool for fostering calm and control in daily life. For many autistic individuals, routines provide predictability and stability in a world that can feel overwhelming. But routines aren't just for neurodivergent individuals – they are universally beneficial. All of us, neurodivergent or not, are wired to thrive on consistency.

The body loves rhythm. Routines – whether it's a nightly skincare ritual, a cup of tea before bed or a favourite playlist – help create a bridge between the stress of the day and the calm needed for restful sleep. In *The Accountant*, Christian Wolff's intense nightly ritual offers him predictability and self-regulation. While it might seem unconventional, it reflects the power of personalisation. When routines are tailored to individual needs, they can become a source of comfort, grounding and renewal.

Touch

Touch is one of the most profound yet often overlooked sensory experiences, especially in discussions of relaxation and sleep. A hug, a gentle hand on the shoulder or even the weight of a pet on your lap can calm the nervous system, releasing oxytocin – the 'bonding hormone' – which reduces stress and promotes relaxation.

Unfortunately, in today's fast-paced world, many people – especially those who live alone – experience a lack of meaningful touch. Days, or even weeks, can pass without a single hug or hand on the back. This deprivation can lead to heightened stress, feelings of isolation and difficulty unwinding.

The good news is that you don't always need someone else to experience the calming benefits of touch. Self-massage, progressive muscle relaxation or even cuddling with soft bedding can provide similar soothing effects. By incorporating intentional moments of touch into your day, you can help your nervous system transition from stress to calm.

Evening skincare relaxation technique

1. Gently wash your face with warm water and your favourite cleanser. As you massage the cleanser into your skin, take slow, deep breaths and focus on the soothing sensation.
2. Apply a toner with a cotton pad, using light, upward strokes. Imagine wiping away the stress of the day along with any remaining impurities.
3. Smooth your favourite moisturiser on to your face and neck, taking your time to massage it in. Pay attention to the texture and fragrance, letting it calm your mind.
4. Use your fingertips to gently massage your face in circular motions, focusing on areas where you hold tension, such as your temples and jawline. Breathe deeply and slowly as you do this.
5. End your skincare routine by taking a few deep breaths, feeling refreshed and ready for a peaceful night's sleep.

The calming power of touch extends beyond daily rituals – it can also enhance sleep. A study in the *Journal of Affective Science* (2022) explored 'sleep touch' among 210 married couples, examining how consensual night-time physical contact influences sleep and emotional wellbeing.[14]

The spectrum of sleep touch varies among couples. For some, it's a close embrace throughout the night; for others, it's a brief touch before retreating to their spaces, or a gentle hand placed on the back. Each form of touch speaks its language of care and presence. The study found that such touch is linked to fewer negative interactions, less stress and a more positive mood upon waking. Interestingly, the impact was more pronounced for husbands, suggesting that touch from their wives contributed to a happier, calmer start to their day. While the effect on sleep quality was less clear, a positive trend indicated that touch enhances sleep. From a polyvagal theory perspective, these interactions activate the safety state, promoting a sense of calm and wellbeing.

Understanding this, we can see that the rituals of touch – whether with a partner, a pet, or even the texture of our bedding – are not just physical interactions. They are deeply tied to our neurobiological state, offering a way to shift our autonomic state into safety and giving us an experience of soothing and comfort as we prepare for sleep. While not everyone has a partner to share touch with, the principle remains the same: gentle contact – whether from a pet, a soft blanket or even the texture of your bedding – can help signal to your body that it's time to let go and rest.

Taste

It might seem strange to think about sensory experiences and sleep together. But when we look at how our daily habits – including eating – impact our sleep, it all makes sense.

Eating can trigger the release of dopamine and endorphins. Stress significantly impacts our food choices, and we know that eating is a common coping mechanism. Studies show that when stressed, we reach for fatty, sugary foods,[15] likely due to high cortisol and insulin levels, and ghrelin also plays a role – exacerbated if you're regularly getting less than five hours a night of sleep or dealing with obesity.[16]

Eating fat- and sugar-laden foods creates a feedback loop that soothes our stress responses and emotions. They aren't called comfort foods for nothing; they help mitigate stress, which explains why we crave them so much during tough times. But there can be a difficult cost.

Stress-related eating often leads to mindless eating, where food is consumed quickly without attention to hunger or fullness cues. Excess weight and poor diet can worsen conditions like sleep apnea, leading to more severe health issues.

Nocturnal eating syndrome or sleep-related eating disorder (SRED) involves episodes of eating during the night, often without full awareness or recollection. Individuals might consume a variety of foods, sometimes including unusual or non-food items. These episodes usually happen when you're partially waking up from deep sleep, often without being fully aware of them.

In his book *The Nocturnal Brain: Nightmares, Neuroscience, and the Secret World of Sleep*, my colleague Professor Guy Leschziner recounts a striking case of a person who, while asleep, ate birdseed – highlighting the serious nature of this disorder and the need for treatment.[17]

Anything food-related can be a minefield of polarising views, but what is often missed in the debate is the importance of social eating, which also offers a valuable opportunity to slow down and connect with others. When did you last take a coffee or lunch break with others instead of sitting alone at your desk, mindlessly eating while glued to the screen?

Everyday communal eating with family and friends is where the real magic happens. Social eating is a universal tradition, even in our fast-food culture. The Big Lunch – a collaboration between the Eden Project and Robin Dunbar, a professor of psychology at the University of Oxford – shows how sharing meals helps us bond, feel happier and stay connected.[18]

Eating together offers immense benefits, not just for nutrition but for our social and emotional wellbeing. For many people (not all, as it can be stressful), sharing a meal strengthens community ties, reinforces relationships and even boosts your health. It's not just eating together – laughing and singing with friends also releases endorphins, making you feel good.

When you eat with others, you tend to eat more slowly, giving your body time to register fullness, potentially leading to eating less. Social interactions naturally slow the pace of eating, helping your brain receive signals from your stomach that you're full. Another way to reduce stress through eating is by practising mindful eating – fully engaging with your food. Notice the colours, smells, textures, flavours and even sounds. Think of it as putting the brakes on your busy day. By slowing down and paying attention to what you're eating, you can make better food choices, avoid overeating and find a bit of calm in your day.

Warm drink before bed?

In the 19th and 20th centuries, Horlicks and other drinks were marketed with claims of promoting sleep, improving digestion and enhancing overall health. These claims were rooted in the ingredients used and the prevailing health beliefs of the time. While some of these claims may have been exaggerated, many of these products remain popular today for their perceived health benefits. Drinks like herbal teas and warm milk, and foods rich in tryptophan are often touted for their sleep-enhancing qualities. Studies have explored the connection between these foods and drinks and sleep, with mixed results. Herbal teas such as chamomile contain apigenin, an antioxidant that may promote sleepiness. Warm milk, with its tryptophan content, is another popular bedtime remedy, though the impact might be more psychological, due to the comfort it brings.[19]

Ultimately, the real power of these foods and drinks might lie in their role as sensory cues. Consuming them consistently before bed helps signal to your body that it's time to prepare for sleep, creating a 'tasty *zeitgeber*' – a taste-based cue that aligns with your internal clock. Through mindful consumption, taste becomes a powerful ally in your quest for a peaceful night.

Smell

Smell is one of our most primal senses, with a direct line to the brain's limbic system, which is responsible for emotions, behaviour and long-term memory. The olfactory system's unique wiring allows certain scents to evoke powerful emotional responses and trigger memories, sometimes buried deep in the subconscious. This direct connection between smell and the brain means that scents can have a profound impact on our psychological state, including our ability to relax and sleep.

For newborns, the connection between smell and sleep begins early. Babies are naturally drawn to their mother's scent, which can have a calming effect, promoting feelings of safety and security that are conducive to sleep. This bond between scent and comfort is deeply ingrained and can continue to influence sleep patterns throughout life.[20] Certain scents are well known for their ability to promote relaxation and improve sleep quality. Aromas like lavender, chamomile and vanilla are particularly effective because they stimulate the release of neurotransmitters such as serotonin and endorphins, which are associated with relaxation and mood stabilisation. Lavender has been extensively studied for its sleep-inducing properties, and research suggests that it may help reduce anxiety and improve sleep quality.

I have worked with many people who lost their sense of smell, also known as anosmia, due to COVID-19. Adapting to life without a sense of smell can be challenging. People rely more on smell than they realise: for cooking, cleaning and personal care. Your olfactory system is unique among the senses because it has a direct pathway to the brain's limbic system, including the amygdala and hippocampus, which are involved in emotion and memory processing. Certain smells can instantly evoke vivid memories or strong emotions – they tell you something that somewhere in your memory bank you already 'know'.[21]

However, not all scents are beneficial for sleep. Unpleasant or invasive odours, such as those from pollution, industrial areas or even certain foods, can disrupt sleep by causing stress and discomfort. For instance, if you live in an area where the air is filled with strong, unpleasant smells, it can be challenging to create a restful environment. These odours can trigger stress responses in the body, making it difficult to relax and fall asleep.

Travel tip

If you travel a lot, taking something with you that carries the aroma of someone familiar can provide a grounding resource, a sensory bridge to home and safety. An interesting study showed that women experienced a stress reduction when exposed to their partner's scent, even without them being present.[22]

Temperature

Temperature plays a big role in sleep. It's a *zeitgeber* – an external cue that helps regulate your body's internal clock. When temperatures rise above or fall below what's normal for you, expect it to affect your sleep. Too hot, and you might feel restless and agitated; too cold, and your muscles can tense up, making you uncomfortable and disrupting your rest.

People often say the best temperature for sleep is around 65°F (18°C), but that's based on research done in cooler, controlled environments. A cooler room helps your body's natural temperature drop, one of the signals it uses to wind down for sleep. This is also why it's not recommended to do intensive exercise right before bed – it raises your core temperature and can get in the way of that cooling process. You need time to cool down and let your body settle into its natural rhythm. In hotter climates, people adapt differently. Take the Spanish siesta, for example – a midday rest during the hottest part of the day, often paired with shorter nighttime sleep. It's a reminder that rest is influenced by where you live and what works for your body.

The takeaway? Sleep isn't about rigid rules or hitting the 'perfect' temperature. It's about creating the right conditions for your body to rest and recharge, wherever you are.

Creating a comfortable sleep environment with moderate temperatures is worth the effort. Using bedding and sleepwear that help regulate your body temperature, like breathable fabrics or temperature-controlled bedding, can make a big difference, as can the use of cooling pads or heated blankets. Separate duvets can be a game-changer for couples – ending the battle over who hogs the duvet and often resulting in the realisation that you need completely different tog weights.

If you're experiencing menopause, your sleep might be especially disrupted by fluctuating body temperatures. One helpful tip is to take a bath or shower before bed. This works because the warm water causes vasodilation, which means your blood vessels widen, increasing blood flow and lowering blood pressure. This process helps your body temperature drop afterwards, aiding relaxation and aligning with your natural sleep rhythm. Understanding and using these body responses can help you fall asleep more easily and enjoy deeper, more restful sleep.

Using temperature to improve sleep

- Taking a warm bath or shower raises your core temperature. When you finish and cool down, the cooling process mimics the natural drop in body temperature before sleep, signalling to your body that it's time to rest.
- Vasodilation, or the widening of blood vessels, increases blood flow to your skin and extremities, helping your body release heat more effectively. This shift of heat from your core leads to a faster and more noticeable drop in body temperature after a bath, helping you feel sleepier.

Relaxation response:
- Warm water relaxes muscles and eases aches, making it easier to fall asleep and improving sleep quality.
- The calming ritual of a bath reduces stress and prepares your mind for sleep.

Circadian rhythm regulation:
- The cooling effect after a warm bath triggers melatonin production, promoting sleep.
- For best results, take a bath one to two hours before bed to align with your natural sleep patterns.

When your living environment is out of your control

Imagine you're trying to create the perfect environment for a good night's sleep. You might think it's all about adjusting the light, setting the right temperature and sticking to a sleep schedule. But what if these things weren't entirely under your control?

Meet Sarah, who lives alone in a large block of flats with a shared heating system. She tells me that she has been trying to improve her sleep by following some advice she found online. 'I have made my bedroom dark, but I hate getting up in the dark when the alarm clock goes off. I feel totally disorientated.' We discuss possible solutions to a common problem – using a light-based alarm clock and opening the curtains as soon as possible. We continue to explore her living space, and Sarah shares that she goes to bed and gets up at the same time every day, but she can't control the temperature – in the winter it's freezing cold and during the summer boiling hot. She finds the vagaries of differing temperatures particularly stressful and it becomes apparent that she is particularly focused on this issue, which has morphed into a dispute with the building's owners.

Unlike a house, where she might have more control, her flat has its quirks. The shared heating system is old, noisy and controlled by the people who manage her block. There is something in the lack of control that is rumbling at the base of Sarah's stress. Curious about it, we explore further. It appears that the issue is triggering a level of anger in Sarah that she feels is controlling her – as she talks about it, she becomes instantly animated, her voice rises and her cheeks flush.

When you face something you can't control or solve, your stress levels can spiral out of control. It's easy to get caught in a cycle of negative thinking – focusing on the problem makes you feel even more powerless, and the stress just keeps piling up. Take Sarah, for example. Her insomnia stems from two factors: the physical discomfort of the temperature and the stress of feeling unable to change the situation. It's a frustrating combination, and it's no wonder she feels stuck.

Sarah's sensory audit

To find a way to feel more in control of her environment, Sarah spent a day noting the sensory inputs in her environment, recording what she saw, heard, smelled, touched and tasted, and thinking about what she could change. This exercise builds awareness, promotes mindfulness, helps identify stress triggers, and highlights what you can do to create a more relaxing and sleep-friendly environment. It's not just about managing your workload or ensuring you get enough sleep; it's also about understanding how your physical surroundings can drain your energy and cause stress.

Time of day	Sensory input	Current situation	Adjustments that Sarah and I discussed
Morning	Sight	Dark from black-out curtains, dim lights	As soon as she wakes, open curtains for sunlight and use a lightbox to increase daylight, a reminder that this will help suppress the release of melatonin, waking you up faster.
	Sound	Alarms, morning news, traffic noise	Use a light-based alarm clock and avoid listening to the news for the first hour of the day.
	Smell	Coffee, body odour, household cleaners	Think about products that have smells you really like rather than mindlessly shopping for home and personal hygiene products. If possible, open the windows.
	Touch	Temperature of home, textures of clothing, bath towels or bedding	Wear clothes that feel good on your skin rather than anything scratchy or uncomfortable.
	Taste	Morning mouth	Toothpaste
	Temperature	Too hot	Close all curtains before leaving home to keep the sun out. Use fans to keep air moving and consider investing in a cooling pad for her bed.
Afternoon	Sight	Computer screens, fluorescent lights	Take breaks from screens, use natural lighting, put a plant on the desk.
	Sound	Office chatter, background music, construction noise	Use noise-cancelling headphones, remove self to quieter spaces.
	Smell	Lunch aromas, air fresheners	Add a lemon-scented pelargonium to her desk, reminding her of her gran's house – a happy place.

Time of day	Sensory input	Current situation	Adjustments that Sarah and I discussed
	Touch	Desk surfaces, chair comfort, room temperature	Ensure ergonomic seating. Get up from desk regularly.
	Taste	Lunch, snacks, beverages	Stop eating at her desk; there isn't anywhere else to eat in the office, so always go outside – she will notice that makes a difference and breaks up the day.
Evening	Sight	TV screens, dim lighting, electronic devices	Changing the table lamps to orange bulbs and turning off ceiling lights give a much nicer feel to the room.
	Sound	TV shows, family conversations, night-time outdoor sounds	Pay attention to the sounds – notice that some sounds are more stimulating than others.
	Smell	Dinner aromas, smell from outside	Use diffusers in a couple of rooms to over-ride external smells.
	Touch	Sofa cushions, evening clothes, bed linens	Use soft, breathable bedding; create a cosy environment.
	Temperature	Too hot	Open all curtains as soon as getting home. Open windows at the back of the flat and all doors, and place a fan in front of the window to move the air through. Consider investing in an air conditioning unit.
		Too cold	Create warm zones in your flat – a corner with cosy blankets and soft lighting in the winter – and electric blanket at night in your bed.

By consciously adjusting your sensory surroundings throughout the day, you feel more in control, which can guide your brain towards relaxation and improve your overall sleep quality.

Light and noise pollution

Sarah's flat is in a city where streetlights shine through her curtains and the sounds of traffic and late-night revellers seep in, no matter what she tries. Globally, stricter lighting and noise regulations and legal recourse are needed to mitigate intrusive environmental factors. Legal cases have addressed excessive lighting and noise, recognising their negative health impacts, such as increased stress, anxiety, hypertension and sleep disorders. Residents living near wind turbines in France experienced significant noise pollution, leading to sleep disturbances, headaches and stress. The persistent low-frequency hum, or 'infra-sound', was particularly intrusive at night. The residents took the case to court.[23] They won, underscoring the importance of considering the health and wellbeing of those living near environmentally intrusive installations.

Proprioception

Proprioception, often called the 'sixth sense', is like an internal GPS; it helps you to 'know' where your body parts are and how they're moving.[24] It is the grounding sense that reassures you, even during sleep, that you are safe and where you need to be. Relying on signals from receptors in the muscles, skin and joints enables smooth and confident movement. Gymnasts rely on proprioception for complex movements, such as somersaults and balancing on beams. A documentary about the US gymnast, Simone Biles, shows her explaining how important this sense is for her to perform well, sharing how when something went wrong with her proprioception, it had a huge impact. She calls this problem the 'twisties', where she loses her sense of direction while twisting in the air, which can be very confusing and danger-ous. The documentary shows how this issue affected her training, performances and mental health. While Simone Biles is an extraor-dinary athlete, we ordinary beings all rely on proprioception in more ways than we might realise. Improving or maintaining our propriocep-tive ability helps maintain quality of life as we age.

Stress can affect proprioception; you might find that you are more clumsy than usual, your coordination is off and you have an overall sense of physical unease. When you go to bed, the feeling that something is off has a knock-on effect. As you settle in, proprioception should help your brain to recognise that you are in a safe, comfortable place, aiding relaxation and making it easier to drift off. If it's out, you will likely find yourself tossing and turning – nothing feels quite right.

How to check your proprioception

Balance test

Stand on one leg with your eyes open for 30 seconds. Then try it with your eyes closed.

What to look for: Your ability to remain steady without swaying or touching the ground with your other foot indicates good proprioception.

Romberg test

Stand with your feet together, arms at your sides and eyes closed for 30 seconds.

What to look for: Minimal swaying or maintaining balance indicates good proprioception.

Ways to improve your proprioception

Balance exercises

- Practise standing on one leg for increasing periods. Use a stability ball for more challenge.
- Incorporate exercises that require balance, like lunges and squats, into your routine.
- Perform some of your exercises with your eyes closed to rely more on proprioceptive feedback rather than visual cues.

Yoga and Pilates: These practices enhance body awareness, balance, and coordination through various poses and controlled movements.

Tai Chi: This form of exercise involves slow, deliberate movements and can improve balance and proprioception as well as reduce stress.

By paying attention to how your body feels as you lie down, you can trigger a sense of relaxation via proprioception. Focus on the weight of the blanket, the texture of the sheets against your skin and the support of the mattress beneath you. This simple act of tuning in to these sensations can help calm your mind and signal to your brain that it's time to wind down.

Think of proprioception as a helpful connection between your body and brain. When you notice these small details, you're giving your brain clear cues that it's safe to relax. It's a way of grounding yourself, reminding you of the comfort and security of your bed and the space around you. This helps shift your nervous system out of the busyness of the day, inviting you to let go and drift into a deep, restful sleep.

Weighted blankets have become a popular tool for enhancing sleep and reducing anxiety. I often recommend them more for afternoon naps as a stress reliever than for bedtime, but it's up to you. The gentle, even pressure mimics a therapeutic technique known as deep touch pressure, which can help the autonomic nervous system feel secure and calm.

Various small studies support the benefits of weighted blankets. A study in the *Journal of Clinical Sleep Medicine* found that participants using weighted blankets reported better sleep, less movement and a greater sense of security.[25] Weighted blankets are not a cure-all – their effectiveness can vary, and for some, the sensation may feel confining rather than comforting.

Proprioception exercises to destress and enhance spatial awareness

These exercises are all helpful in reducing stress and increasing your spatial awareness. There is something compelling about using your body to change your emotional state. We often move repetitively on the same planes, so challenging this habit is helpful to remind your body of its adaptability and strength, and to reduce injury.

Weightbearing activity

- Find a clear space where you can move freely. Get down on all fours and crawl slowly around the area for 2–3 minutes. Focus on the movement of your hands and knees, feeling the pressure on your joints.

Resistance activities

- Use a resistance band or a towel. Hold each end and pull as if trying to stretch it as far as possible. Hold for 10 seconds, then relax. Repeat this five times.
- Alternatively, push against a wall with both hands, leaning your weight into it for 10 seconds, then relax. Repeat five times. This can also be useful for reducing feelings of frustration or anger.

Heavy lifting

- Pick up a few heavy books or other weighted objects. Walk around the room, focusing on how the weight feels in your arms and the muscles working to carry the load. Do this for 2–3 minutes.

Oral activities

- Chew a piece of gum slowly, paying attention to the movement of your jaw. This can be useful if you have bruxism, to give the temporal mandibular joint – the most powerful joint in the body – some alternative movement.

- Blow bubbles with a bubble solution, concentrating on your breath and the formation of the bubbles.

Deep pressure
- Give yourself a tight hug, wrapping your arms around your body and squeezing gently but firmly. Hold for 10–15 seconds, then release. Repeat three times. If you have a partner or a family member who you trust, maybe ask them for a hug.

Do nothing to get more

I find it fascinating that we've reached a point where we need a concept – or even a trend – to give ourselves permission to do nothing. It says so much about how deeply we've bought into the idea that being busy equals being valuable. But just existing, with no purpose or goal, already has a name – *niksen*.[26]

What makes it even more intriguing is where *niksen* comes from. The Netherlands, a country shaped by its Calvinistic heritage that holds productivity and hard work as core values. In such a context, *niksen* feels rebellious. It's like saying, 'No, I don't have to keep doing. I can just be.'

But here's the question: why do you need permission to stop? To let go? What does it say about the world we live in that doing nothing feels unnatural – or even wrong? When you pause and let yourself just be, however, you're not really doing nothing. You're resetting, giving your mind and body space to process, to breathe. Maybe that's why *niksen* feels so sticky. It's not just about the practice itself – it's about what it challenges in a world that's forgotten how to simply exist.

Sitting quietly with your thoughts can feel like a revolutionary act of self-discovery. It's not about being lazy; it's about finding moments of stillness and relaxation amid all the hustle and bustle. *Niksen* lets you tune in to your true desires and instincts, free from societal expectations and pressures. It aims to create space for relaxation and mental rest, and allows the mind to wander freely, promoting creativity and reducing stress.

You don't need to make drastic changes to embrace *niksen*. It can be as simple as gazing out of the window, sitting quietly with a cup of tea or lying down without the goal of sleeping. The essence lies in choosing to do nothing, creating a deliberate pause in the busyness of life. Unlike mindfulness, which may feel structured or overly engaging for some, *niksen* is about effortless idleness and spontaneous relaxation. While mindfulness requires focus and discipline, *niksen* invites you to simply let go. Both can work together, offering different routes to mental clarity and a sense of calm.

How to practise *niksen*

1. Find a comfortable spot where you won't be disturbed.
2. Allow yourself to sit or lie down without any specific goal.
3. Let your mind wander freely without trying to focus on anything in particular.
4. Embrace the stillness and enjoy the act of doing nothing.

Just breathe

Quite often, when working with someone, I might need to remind them to breathe. Just check in with yourself right now: are you breathing? Where is your breath? Is it high up in your chest or are you breathing down into your belly? If you are stressed or have experienced a lot of trauma, it is normal (though it might be quite surprising to realise) just how much you might be holding your breath or not breathing fully.

Need to relax?

Try this simple exercise:

- Close your eyes.
- Breathe in slowly.

- Breathe out for longer than you took to breathe in.
- Repeat for five minutes.

This activates your parasympathetic nervous system, helping you calm down and clear your mind. Just five minutes can make a big difference! And you can do it as often as you like.

It seems that the ancient yogis were on to something. They may not have understood biology, but the ancient practice of yoga was all about the preparation to breathe. Breathwork can provide a mental pause button. This brief pause allows a more measured response to thoughts and stimuli rather than getting caught in a whirlwind of circular thinking – changing your breath can change your emotional state.[27]

When we inhale, our heart rate increases, and as we exhale, it starts to slow down. Research indicates that deep belly breathing activates the part of the nervous system that helps reduce stress and promotes relaxation.[28] Additionally, reports have shown that individuals with a history of trauma often exhibit disrupted breathing patterns, which, while logical, can unfortunately make symptoms of anxiety and stress worse.[29] Imagine something startles you; you are likely to hold your breath momentarily. This startle reflex is an automatic response to sudden stimuli, involving a brief stop in breathing, increased heartbeat and muscle tension.

Often, when working with people, I carefully explain and then show the technique so that they can go away and experiment with it until they feel comfortable enough for us to work on it together. It can feel weird to sit one-on-one in a room with someone, just breathing! I have been studying and practising breathwork for many years. I recall being stunned by a teacher who shared how breathing rates have more than doubled over the last 100 years; decades ago, people typically breathed at a rate of five to six breaths per minute.[30] That rate has nearly doubled to 12–15 breaths per minute.[31] There are likely many reasons for this change, including stress and environmental issues, but the implications are enormous. Rapid breathing perpetuates our stress responses, increasing reactivity, anxiety and irritability, making hair-trigger reactions the norm, and eroding our ability to pause and thoughtfully consider the space between stimulus and response.

The science of breathwork

Breathing is something you do over 20,000 times a day without thinking about it. But when done mindfully, it can become a powerful tool to calm your mind, reduce stress and improve sleep. Think of breathwork as a reset button that is always accessible to you. The science behind it shows how truly powerful conscious breathing can be.

When you inhale, it's like pressing the accelerator pedal – it activates and energises your body. On the other hand, the act of exhaling is what calms you. When you take rapid, shallow breaths, you can trigger hyperventilation, which activates the sympathetic nervous system – the part of the body that's preparing for fight-or-flight, leaving you feeling wired or anxious.

The breathing technique advocated by Wim Hof, often called the 'Wim Hof Method', involves cycles of deep, rapid breathing, followed by breath-holding. It's designed to increase oxygen levels in the body, stimulate the nervous system, and create a sense of heightened energy and focus.

While this method has many benefits – such as boosting energy, improving focus and even helping with stress management – it's not the best choice right before bed. Instead, when you focus on slow, deliberate exhalation, you engage the parasympathetic nervous system – the body's 'rest-and-digest' state – via the vagus nerve. This is activated by the diaphragm, the large muscle under the rib cage. In short, slow breathing signals to your body that it's safe to relax.

You might be sceptical about the calming power of breath, thinking it sounds a bit too easy. However, the mechanism is relatively straightforward. It's handy because it combines both automatic and voluntary control of breathing, making it an effective tool for managing anxiety and promoting a sense of calm in real-life situations. The autonomic nervous system, which operates without conscious effort, regulates bodily functions like heart, digestion and respiration, keeping them in sync. When stressed, everything speeds up; when calm, everything slows down. Although we can't directly command our heart to slow down just by thinking about it, breathing is unique because it's both automatic and under our control, making it a powerful tool.

As you drop into the first stage of NREM sleep, the brain shifts from a beta state – where you probably are right now – into alpha, then theta.

We can enter the theta state by slowing down breathing deliberately. This is why meditation can feel so relaxing: slowing your breath helps shift your brain into a different state. When you're in the theta state, your brainwaves slow to frequencies of between 4 and 8 Hz. This state is great for creativity, intuition and processing memories.

Slow, deep breaths communicate to your body that you are safe, not in immediate danger, and it's OK to relax. This simple act gives the body permission to lower its defences and calm down. Breathwork has been shown to affect cognitive function and mental health profoundly. Research suggests that regular breathwork practices can improve attention, concentration and cognitive performance, while also reducing symptoms of anxiety and depression. By incorporating breathwork into your day, you have a powerful tool to put the brakes on and slow everything down. Best of all, like light, breathing is free! A beautiful addition to working with the breath is the simple reminder to smile – then breathe. I picked up this little gem from a Qigong teacher, and it's become a cornerstone of my own breathwork practice.

Before we dive into different techniques, here's a gentle reminder: please approach breathwork and meditation mindfully. Many people feel frustrated when mental health professionals suggest mindfulness and breathwork as cure-alls – they aren't for everyone. If you find these practices stressful, maybe seek a teacher or a class to support you. If you have a specific mental health condition like PTSD or bipolar disorder, it's especially important to understand the potential risks and proceed with care. It is also not advised for those with chronic obstructive pulmonary disease (COPD), asthma or for those who are pregnant. These practices are powerful, so be gentle with yourself as you explore these deeper states of consciousness. Respect your own pace and needs.

Breathing techniques

Waking up in the middle of the night with a racing heart or sense of panic can be unsettling. In these moments, breathwork can help calm your nervous system. Here's how you can defuse panic with your breath (these are all *different* breathing techniques experiment, so choose the one(s) that works best for you).

Focus on the exhale

When panic hits, your breaths may become short and shallow. Start by focusing on lengthening your exhale, as this helps signal to your body that you're safe. Try to make your exhale longer than your inhale, even if it's just by a few seconds.

Popularised by Dr Andrew Huberman, this technique was initially discovered in the 1930s and has been further researched by scientists like Professor Jack Feldman and Mark Krasnow. It's one of the quickest ways to calm yourself, especially in moments of high stress.

The physiological sigh

1. One deep inhale through the nose.
2. One short inhale to top up.
3. One long exhale to empty lungs.

Just 1–3 cycles emphasising the out-breath will slow your heart rate and relax you in real-time.

Diaphragmatic breathing (or belly breathing)

1. Sit or lie down comfortably.
2. Place one hand on your chest and the other on your abdomen.
3. Inhale slowly and deeply through your nose, allowing your abdomen to rise (your chest should remain relatively still).
4. Exhale slowly and thoroughly through your mouth or nose.

Continue for 5–10 minutes, or as long as feels comfortable.

4–7–8 breathing

1. Inhale quietly through your nose for 4 seconds.
2. Hold your breath for 7 seconds.
3. Exhale forcefully through your mouth, pursing your lips and making a whooshing sound, for 8 seconds.

This completes one cycle. Repeat for four cycles initially, and with practice, you can increase to eight cycles.

Box breathing (or square breathing)
1. Inhale for a count of 4.
2. Hold your breath for a count of 4.
3. Exhale for a count of 4.
4. Hold your breath again for a count of 4.
5. Repeat this pattern several times.

Integrating breathwork throughout your day
- Morning routine: start your day with 5–10 minutes of breathwork to immediately slow stress down.
- Take a few moments for mindful breathing before transitioning from one task or meeting to the next.
- Use phone reminders to prompt you to take 1–2 minutes of deep breathing every couple of hours.
- Red traffic lights are perfect places to breathe for a bit.
- When overwhelmed or stressed, step away and practise a few minutes of breathwork.
- End your day with breathwork to help transition from work to relaxation or before bedtime to improve sleep.

The struggle of chronic pain and sleep

Living with chronic pain can feel like an endless battle, especially when it comes to getting a good night's sleep. Pain doesn't just make it hard to fall asleep – it wakes you up throughout the night, trapping you in a cycle where poor sleep makes the pain worse, and pain makes it hard to sleep.

After taking medical retirement from the military due to complex health problems, sleep became a distant dream for Mathis. When asked about it, he responded, 'Sleeping? It's more like waging war. I dread bedtime. When I have a flare of my fibromyalgia, it feels like every joint is on fire. I toss and turn, and when I do manage to fall asleep, the pain wakes me up.'

Chronic pain can make the night seem endless, a battleground rather than a place of rest. When asked if his sleep is ever restful, Mathis shook his head. 'I wake up feeling more exhausted, if that's even possible.' This fragmented sleep means he misses out on the deep, restorative stages.

People with conditions like fibromyalgia, arthritis and neuropathy frequently experience disruptions in their sleep stages. Chronic pain disrupts this pattern, causing frequent awakenings and preventing restorative sleep. Combining pain management strategies, good sleep routines and targeted interventions can help break the cycle. Managing chronic pain is an arduous journey, requiring patience and resilience.

Pacing – managing energy levels

'Pacing' means breaking down the 24 hours of your day into smaller, manageable tasks balanced with regular rest periods, helping to avoid overexertion and reduce painful flare-ups. I often guide clients through this process using the '24 hours in a day' exercise from Chapter Three. Rest, here, is an active, intentional practice. When incorporated regularly, it can reduce inflammation, restore energy and aid in pain management.

Energy pacing, aligned with your circadian rhythms and chronotype, allows you to plan your activities around natural peaks and dips in energy. A structured day, with planned rest breaks, adds predictability, making life feel more manageable and reducing anxiety.

Relaxation techniques like breathwork and gentle exercise, such as swimming (which reduces pressure on the body through buoyancy), are also important tools. However, the true challenge lies in acceptance – acknowledging the presence of pain without constantly battling against it. This shift in mindset, which may require support from a therapist, can transform your relationship with discomfort.

Rather than 'fighting' illness, which activates the stress response, acceptance allows for a more peaceful approach. This journey isn't easy, but it ultimately brings a kind of peace – not from eliminating difficulties, but from changing how we relate to them.

Effective energy pacing

Stay flexible: listen to your body and adjust your schedule as needed.

Prioritise tasks: focus on high-priority tasks during peak times and less critical tasks during low-energy periods.

Mindfulness and relaxation: incorporate mindfulness practices like meditation or deep breathing exercises to manage stress and maintain focus.

Managing sleep with chronic pain also requires rethinking how your sleep works. Polyphasic sleep, the practice of breaking sleep into shorter periods throughout the day, and anchor sleep, which centres on a core night's sleep supplemented by naps, offer alternative approaches. Both acknowledge the body's natural rhythms and limitations, allowing rest to happen in a more fluid, less constrained way. Pain or no pain, there's no need to keep pushing for what the body cannot deliver. Understanding and accepting these softer approaches to sleep involves fostering a kinder relationship with your body, acknowledging limitations and working within boundaries to support health and wellbeing.

This shift in perspective requires you to accept that sleep might come in shorter, more fragmented bursts. By recognising this and planning for it, you can create a sleep strategy that aligns with your body's needs and pain patterns. For instance, you might find that incorporating short naps or rest periods into your day can help alleviate the pressure to achieve all your rest in one go, ultimately leading to better overall sleep quality and pain management.

Much like other aspects of living with chronic pain, sleep should be thoughtfully structured and integrated into your rest and recovery plan. This requires the same level of attention and adaptation as your daily activities and pacing strategies. While it can be disheartening to invest effort in these adjustments, it is a vital part of fostering a compassionate relationship with your body. Acknowledging the limitations imposed by chronic pain and working within those boundaries will help you find a rhythm that supports your health and wellbeing.

Summary

Our pursuit of restful sleep is not merely the absence of wakefulness but an intricate blend of sensory experiences. The whispers of a loved one's voice, the soothing touch of a soft blanket, the calming associations of a favourite scent – these sensory encounters are not just passive experiences but active participants in our nightly ritual of letting go of the day.

The pathway towards sound sleep is also an inward journey. It is a recognition that our bodies are not isolated mechanisms but interconnected systems where the mind, body and environment come together to create the conditions for rest. By paying attention to our sensory world, we can make a deeper connection to ourselves and our surroundings – and become more grounded in a world that seems to be spinning ever faster.

Consider Jenna, whose overwhelming sensory experiences had become nightly adversaries. She began reclaiming her nights through mindful engagement with her environment and guided practices. The simple exercise of focusing on her hand, of observing and feeling without judgement, became a gateway to calm. This seemingly mundane practice illuminated a profound truth: within us lies the capacity to shape our sensory world, to transform it from a source of distress into a place of quiet calm.

Actionable steps

- Spend at least 20 minutes outdoors each morning to expose yourself to natural light. If sunlight is scarce, consider using a light therapy lamp.
- Design your bedroom to be a haven for sleep. Keep it cool, dark and quiet. Invest in comfortable bedding and consider using blackout curtains, earplugs or white noise machines as needed.
- Establish a 'digital sunset' by turning off electronic devices at least an hour before bedtime. If necessary, use blue light filters or apps that adjust the screen's colour temperature.

- Set aside time each day to sit quietly without any agenda. Allow your mind to wander without focusing on specific thoughts or tasks.
- Find sensory experiences that uniquely relax you – whether it's humming, listening to specific music genres, or engaging in tactile activities like knitting or gentle self-massage.
- Practise breathing exercises like diaphragmatic breathing, the physiological sigh or box breathing several times a day.
- Identify situations that trigger sensory overload and develop strategies to mitigate them, such as taking breaks from crowded places, adjusting lighting or using sensory tools like stress balls.
- Use strategies like the 20-20-20 rule for eye strain, noise-cancelling headphones for loud environments or calming scents in your workspace.
- Explore exercises that enhance body awareness, such as yoga, tai chi or balance training. Simple practices like standing on one leg can improve proprioception.
- Recognise that improving sleep is a gradual process. Celebrate small victories and be gentle with yourself if progress feels slow.

CHAPTER SEVEN

Integrating sleep disorders across the lifespan

As a psychotherapist, I encounter many clients who struggle with issues that may be linked to sleep disorders. When in doubt, I always refer them to medical professionals for a formal diagnosis before continuing our work.

I've added this chapter on sleep disorders because understanding what might be happening can empower you to gather evidence before seeing your GP.

From a psychological perspective, there's often a chicken-and-egg situation when it comes to sleep and mental health. It's not always clear whether the sleep issue came first and led to psychological challenges, or if underlying psychological issues are disrupting sleep. This makes it all the more important to understand the potential connections between your sleep patterns and your overall wellbeing.

Sleep is a non-negotiable biological process essential for cognitive function, mood regulation, immune function and cellular repair. However, how you experience sleep is influenced by factors like age, gender, lifestyle and environment. For example, young children require more sleep, while older adults often experience lighter and shorter sleep periods.[1] Gender differences also play a role, with women more likely to experience insomnia due to hormonal changes during menstruation, pregnancy and menopause.[2] Lifestyle factors like work schedules and stress levels also significantly impact sleep patterns, with shift work notably disrupting circadian rhythms.[3]

Remember, your sleep needs and natural sleep preferences – your chronotype (whether you're a 'morning lark' or 'night owl') – shift over time, making everyone's sleep experience unique. This chapter aims to provide you with insight – not to diagnose, but to help you better understand your sleep and take informed steps when seeking help.

Sleep disorders

The hungry beast that is insomnia

Imagine lying in bed, staring at the ceiling, waiting for sleep to come. Everyone experiences this occasionally, but for some, it's a nightly battle. Insomnia becomes a disorder when it meets certain criteria: difficulty falling asleep, staying asleep or feeling refreshed, despite having enough time and the right environment to sleep; daytime issues arising as a consequence; and this all occurring at least three times a week for over a month.

Insomnia is common, comes in different guises and affects 10–30 per cent of people worldwide.[4] It is thought to be linked to hyperarousal, which means being in a state of heightened alertness throughout the day and night. This can be due to cognitive factors (worrying about sleep) and physiological factors (increased metabolic rate, heart rate and stress hormone levels). These factors make it harder to fall and stay asleep. It often shows up with other conditions – there is something of the chicken and the egg about it, in that it is often unclear whether insomnia causes depression and anxiety, or vice versa. However, we do know that insomnia may increase the risk of developing depression and treating it can improve outcomes for those with depression. Conditions like sleep apnea or RLS can also interfere. Cognitive behavioural therapy for insomnia (CBT-I) is highly effective, focusing on the thoughts and behaviours that perpetuate insomnia. You can access it online, in person or from a book.

Insomnia varies greatly from person to person. While it often resolves on its own, chronic insomnia can severely impact daily life. Unrealistic expectations about sleep can worsen insomnia, so accurately assessing sleep patterns can help, as can addressing any underlying health issues or medication side effects – this can include over-the-counter remedies too. I have seen an alarming number of issues causes by excessive use of stimulants in supplement form. Start with a gradual approach. The advice in Chapter One is a good first step. Remember, many behaviours around insomnia are hard to change, but with time *they are* entirely changeable. Be gentle with yourself and allow yourself that time.

Insomnia is like a hungry beast, quickly becoming dominant. Trying to solve it is logical, but often these efforts keep it alive. The '3 Ps' model explains its persistence: predisposing factors (like family history or being a natural worrier), precipitating factors (like stress or life changes) and perpetuating factors (like poor sleep habits).

Perpetuating factors are the behaviours we adopt to cope with poor sleep that worsen the problem. These include things like going to bed too early and staying in bed for too long. Taking daytime naps means you spend more of your sleep pressure, diluting what's available by the time you come to go to bed. Insomnia becomes the dominant factor, and you start to cancel plans due to poor sleep and get very rigid about routines and timing. These actions lead to more time in bed worrying, thus making it worse.

Breaking the cycle

If you have been struggling with insomnia for a while, you might be prescribed sleeping pills as a short-term solution, but they won't fix the long-term problem. You will likely have more success if you can access CBT-I. Too often, people take medication long-term, though there are specific cases where this might be appropriate – especially if you are significantly depressed or are highly anxious and unable to cope. That is for your doctor to decide. Medications can be useful if you know you have them – a psychological crutch – but how you use them can become a problem. Sleeping pills, especially taken in the middle of the night, can become problematic – leading to grogginess and poor cognitive function the next day. They can also lead to self-recrimination – where you criticise yourself for taking them, which only increases stress. Instead of relying on pills, focus on improving sleep habits and managing stress.

CBT-I is often the first line of treatment recommended by sleep specialists because it's not just about managing symptoms; it's about addressing the root causes of your sleep difficulties.

CBT-I works by helping you change the thoughts and behaviours that might be keeping you awake at night. For example, if you find yourself lying in bed, wide awake, worrying about how you'll function the next day, CBT-I teaches you strategies to manage those racing thoughts. It also helps you establish healthier sleep habits, like going to bed and waking up at the same time each day, creating a calming pre-sleep routine and limiting activities in bed that aren't sleep-related.

One of the great things about CBT-I is that it's a practical, structured approach. You work through specific techniques, such as sleep restriction, which helps you spend only the necessary amount of time in bed, and stimulus control, which retrains your brain to associate the bed with sleep rather than wakefulness. Research shows that CBT-I can significantly improve sleep quality for most people with insomnia, and the benefits often last well beyond the treatment period. Unlike sleeping pills, which can sometimes be a short-term fix, CBT-I equips you with tools you can use for the rest of your life to maintain good sleep.

Rebound insomnia

Rebound insomnia can occur when you stop taking sleep medications, especially after long-term use, and can be distressing if you're not prepared for it. This type of insomnia can be even worse than the initial sleep problems the medication was intended to treat.

To manage rebound insomnia effectively, work on building the confidence and understanding that you *can* sleep naturally. When I work with clients on this issue, a significant part of the process is building the scaffolding to face the night when it gets tough. This involves having a plan and the necessary tools in place to ride out the storm. By preparing in advance, you can reduce anxiety and improve your chances of maintaining good sleep habits, even without medication.

- **Tapering off medication:** gradually reduce your dosage with the guidance of a healthcare provider. This process helps your body adjust to the change and reduces the likelihood of severe rebound insomnia.
- **Develop a toolbox of strategies that you can rely on if you struggle to sleep or are having issues with daytime alertness.** These might include relaxation techniques, light exposure, a consistent bedtime routine and activities that promote calmness.

- **Mindset and confidence:** reinforce your belief in your ability to sleep without medication. This might include cognitive-behavioural strategies to address anxiety about sleep and improve your overall sleep behaviours.
- **Professional support:** engage with a sleep specialist or therapist who can provide tailored advice and support throughout the process. They can help you develop and stick to a plan, ensuring that you have the right tools to manage your sleep.
- **Remember, your body knows how to sleep.**

Hypersomnia

Hypersomnia and insomnia are two sides of the same coin. Both are sleep disorders impacting the regulation of sleep but manifesting in opposite symptoms: one involves insufficient sleep, and the other involves excessive sleepiness. While hypersomnia can be a symptom of neurological issues, it is still categorised under sleep disorders due to its primary effect on sleep patterns.

Instead of struggling to sleep, you might find yourself sleeping excessively – sometimes ten hours or more each night – and still feel unrefreshed. People with hypersomnia (excessive daytime sleepiness) often experience overwhelming daytime sleepiness, leading them to take long naps during the day, which unfortunately doesn't alleviate the fatigue. Idiopathic hypersomnia is when someone sleeps for long periods and wakes up feeling confused or irritable (known as sleep inertia) and not refreshed. Despite getting what seems like enough sleep, hypersomnia sufferers are often battling persistent drowsiness, which can severely impact daily life, making it difficult to work, study or even enjoy social activities.

People with hypersomnia sleep disorders may have other symptoms that affect their sleep and their ability to function during the day. They often live without a correct diagnosis for a long time. They may blame themselves and struggle to keep up with work, studies and relationships. If you suspect you may have this, you need to see your GP, who will refer you to a neurologist for further investigation.

Hypersomnia sleep disorders include:

- Idiopathic hypersomnia
- Narcolepsy type 2 (without cataplexy)
- Narcolepsy type 1 (with cataplexy)
- Kleine-Levin syndrome (KLS)
- Hypersomnia and narcolepsy associated with other disorders[5]

Understanding different types of sleep apnea and their implications

Sleep apnea wears several masks, and understanding them can help us address the issue more effectively:

- **Obstructive sleep apnea (OSA):** the most common form of sleep apnea. It occurs when the muscles in the throat relax excessively during sleep, causing a partial or complete blockage of the airway. This obstruction results in brief interruptions in breathing, effectively leading to moments of suffocation. These episodes can deprive the brain of essential oxygen, potentially causing long-term cognitive and health issues. Individuals with certain craniofacial anomalies, such as a recessed jaw or enlarged tonsils, are more prone to developing OSA. Structural issues can narrow the airway, making it more susceptible to obstruction during sleep.
- **Central sleep apnea (CSA):** unlike OSA, CSA is a disorder where breathing stops due to a lack of respiratory effort. This occurs because the brain fails to send appropriate signals to the muscles that control breathing. CSA can be caused by medical conditions affecting the brainstem, such as heart failure, stroke or certain medications. It is less common than OSA but equally important to diagnose and treat.
- **Mixed sleep apnea:** Also known as complex sleep apnea, this condition is a combination of both obstructive and central sleep apnea. It often starts as OSA, but upon treatment with CPAP (continuous positive airway pressure) therapy, the central apneas become apparent.
- **Upper airway resistance syndrome (UARS):** UARS is another common form of sleep-disordered breathing, characterised by

increased resistance to airflow in the upper airway. Unlike OSA, which involves complete or partial obstructions, UARS results in frequent arousals and fragmented sleep due to the increased effort to breathe against the resistance. Both OSA and UARS can be influenced by anatomical factors, such as the structure of the jaw, palate and airway, as well as body weight and fat distribution.

AHI (apnea-hypopnea index) is a key measure for diagnosing sleep apnea, but it's not the only indicator. Other important metrics include the oxygen desaturation index (ODI), which tracks drops in blood oxygen, and the respiratory disturbance index (RDI), which accounts for all sleep disruptions. Additionally, sleep architecture, clinical symptoms and co-morbid conditions are considered. Comprehensive sleep studies (polysomnography) provide detailed insights beyond AHI, offering a fuller picture of the patient's sleep health.

I mentioned sleep apnea briefly on page 104 when discussing food and alcohol, but it's important to note that sleep apnea is not solely caused by weight issues. While weight can be a factor, sleep apnea and other sleep-disordered breathing conditions like upper airway resistance syndrome (UARS) can affect individuals of all body types.[6] UARS is characterised by increased resistance to airflow due to a narrowing of the upper airway, leading to sleep disruptions without complete obstruction. One of the main causes of snoring and these sleep disorders is the relaxation of the lower jaw and surrounding tissues during sleep, which causes the airway to narrow or vibrate. This can obstruct airflow, leading to reduced oxygen intake, frequent arousals from sleep, and gasping. While weight loss, avoiding alcohol and nicotine, and changing sleep position (especially avoiding sleeping on your back) are common recommendations, there are other solutions as well. For example, sewing tennis balls into the back of nightwear can encourage side sleeping, although its effectiveness varies. There are also specialised positional sleep retraining devices available online that may help.

If you're diagnosed with sleep apnea, one potential treatment is the use of mandibular advancement devices (MADs). These devices gently move your lower jaw forward while you sleep, helping to keep your airway open and prevent it from collapsing. This can significantly reduce snoring and improve your night-time breathing. However, MADs must be considered only after a thorough sleep study and under the guidance of a sleep specialist rather than relying solely on a dentist's initial recommendation.

Alternatively, you may be prescribed positive airway pressure (PAP) therapy, which includes machines like CPAP and APAP. Both treat obstructive sleep apnea but differ in how they deliver air pressure. CPAP provides a constant, fixed pressure, while APAP automatically adjusts the pressure based on your breathing needs throughout the night. These machines keep your airway open by delivering airflow through a mask, improving your sleep, overall health and relationships, as they can dramatically reduce snoring and daytime fatigue.

It's really common for people to find these machines uncomfortable or even a bit claustrophobic at first. Many people need to try a few different masks before they find one that fits well and feels comfortable. Don't worry if it takes some trial and error – finding the right fit can make a big difference in sticking with the treatment and getting the full benefits. Just remember, you're not alone in this, and with a little patience, you're likely to find an option that works for you.

Several studies have found that obstructive sleep apnea (OSA) is linked to a higher chance of early death.[7] The serious implications of untreated sleep apnea include reduced oxygen supply to the brain and other vital organs, escalating the risk of severe health issues like hypertension, heart disease, stroke and type 2 diabetes. These conditions highlight the critical nature of diagnosing and effectively managing sleep apnea. Moreover, sleep apnea is not confined to any specific demographic. It can affect individuals of any gender, age or body type, debunking the myth that it is solely a condition affecting overweight, middle-aged men.

Recent studies indicate that up to 80 per cent of sleep apnea cases remain undiagnosed in the UK,[8] underscoring the vast underestimation of this condition's prevalence, and the urgent need for increased awareness and diagnostic efforts. Getting a diagnosis and treatment for sleep apnea may not just save your marriage; it could also save your life!

STOP-Bang questionnaire

If you're concerned that you might have sleep apnea, one of the first steps you can take is to complete an online questionnaire, such as the STOP-Bang questionnaire. Simply search for 'STOP-Bang questionnaire' or 'sleep apnea questionnaire' in your preferred search engine. This will lead you to various websites that offer the questionnaire for free. It is a simple and widely used screening tool that assesses your risk for obstructive sleep apnea (OSA). The acronym 'STOP-Bang'[9] stands for:

- **S**noring: Do you snore loudly (louder than talking or loud enough to be heard through closed doors)?
- **T**ired: Do you often feel tired, fatigued or sleepy during the daytime?
- **O**bserved: Has anyone observed you stop breathing during your sleep?
- **P**ressure: Do you have or are you being treated for high blood pressure?

and

- **B**ody Mass Index (BMI): Is your BMI more than 35 kg/m^2?
- **A**ge: Are you older than 50 years?
- **N**eck circumference: Is your neck circumference greater than 40 cm (16 inches)?
- **G**ender: Are you male?

Scoring high on this questionnaire suggests a higher risk for sleep apnea and indicates that you should consider seeking a professional evaluation.

You think you have a sleep disorder: what next?

Maybe you're struggling with persistent daytime fatigue, or your partner has commented on your loud snoring or restless movements at night. Perhaps you frequently wake up in the early hours, unable to drift back to sleep. Recognising these symptoms is an important first step, but figuring out what to do next can feel overwhelming, especially when the causes of sleep disturbances are so varied.

Your sleep challenges might be influenced by your current phase of life. For instance, young adults often struggle with circadian misalignment due to lifestyle pressures, while midlife brings its own challenges, such as work stress or caring responsibilities. Later in life, health conditions or changes in sleep architecture can play a role. Understanding how life stages interact with sleep can provide valuable clues to what might be causing your difficulties.

The first practical step, no matter your age or situation, is to evaluate your daily routines and habits. Start with a sleep diary – documenting your bedtime and wake-up time, noting any night-time awakenings and recording details about your day-to-day activities, such as exercise, diet and stress levels – for a couple of weeks. This simple exercise can be incredibly illuminating, helping you identify patterns or triggers specific to your life stage and circumstances.

How sleep needs and chronotypes change – from newborns to young adults

While I don't work with children or those under 18, I do work with many new parents. A baby's arrival changes everything, and time can feel like it's slipping into an entirely new rhythm. How you and your partner share childcare, manage the mental load, and the kind of support you receive from family and friends all play a huge role in your stress levels and sleep. And, of course, everyone will have an opinion on how you're handling it!

Not everyone has the advantage of a partner or a strong support network, which can make this already challenging time even harder.

Balancing the demands of parenting with responsibilities like paying bills only adds to the stress. Concerns about your baby's health, adjusting to new roles and the sheer exhaustion of caring for a newborn can make it difficult to get the rest you need. Postpartum depression and anxiety are also common and can further disrupt sleep, creating a cycle that's tough to break.

Newborns and infants

Newborns (0–3 months)	As a new parent, it's helpful to know that newborns need a lot of sleep – about 14 to 17 hours each day. But unlike adults, they don't follow a regular sleep–wake cycle yet. They sleep in short bursts throughout the day and night because their tiny bodies haven't figured out the difference between day and night. It usually takes until they're about three to four months old for their internal clock to start getting in sync. While this fragmented sleep pattern is completely normal and essential for their brain development and growth,[10] I know it can be tough on you. The good news is that you can gently help shape your baby's sleep by exposing them to natural daylight, keeping feeding times consistent and establishing a calming bedtime routine.
Infants (4–11 months)	During this time, you might also start to see early signs of their natural sleep preferences, or what we call a chronotype. This is basically whether your baby is more of a morning lark or a night owl in the making! These emerging patterns are influenced by regular exposure to natural light and having consistent daily routines![11] So, keeping a steady schedule and letting in that sunlight during the day can really help guide their sleep patterns as they grow.

You've probably heard the advice to 'sleep when your baby sleeps,' and while it's well-intentioned, I've lost count of how many new parents tell me how unrealistic and frustrating that suggestion can be. Between other responsibilities and your own body's natural rhythm, it's not always that simple. But when you can, sneaking in naps and finding moments to rest can make a big difference.

I know this part can be really irritating to hear, especially when you're already feeling overwhelmed. It can feel like just one more thing to worry about. But this is often where the real work is needed in therapy. Babies are incredibly in tune with the emotions of the people around them – it's how they're wired to survive. Even at a very young age, they can pick up on different facial expressions and tones of voice and will react accordingly.[12] They often mirror what they see and feel, so if you're calm, they're more likely to be calm, and if you're stressed, well, they pick up on that too. It's not about being perfect or never feeling stressed – because, let's face it, that's impossible. It's about being aware of how your emotions can affect your baby and them learning how you manage your stress – then as they grow, they know it's OK to be stressed as they know how to deal with it.

I see first-hand the profound impact that societal support, or the lack thereof, has on pregnant women and new parents. I feel strongly about this issue because the evidence is clear: investing in this critical stage of life yields significant long-term benefits. Regular prenatal care reduces complications during pregnancy and childbirth, leading to healthier outcomes for mother and child. Postnatal support, including mental health services and parenting education, further enhances health outcomes for the entire family.[13]

Healthier parents and children mean a more productive workforce. Early-childhood programmes boost cognitive and social development, setting children up for success. The ripple effects are enormous, reducing long-term healthcare costs and social inequalities. Yet, despite this evidence, our political system remains short-sighted. Policymakers often focus on short-term gains and overlook the substantial long-term advantages of supporting pregnant women and new parents. This short-sightedness is not just a political failing; it's a societal one.

I work with parents struggling under the weight of inadequate support every day. They face preventable health issues, mental health challenges and developmental concerns with their children that could have been mitigated with the right early interventions. It's frustrating because we know what works; we know that investing in these early stages of life pays off exponentially, but the political will to make these necessary investments is often lacking. As a new parent, you may feel overwhelmed, sleep-deprived and responsible for this new life. It's not easy, and seeking out support – while it might feel like another thing 'to do' – can pay dividends over time.

Toddlerhood and beyond

Toddlers (1–2 years)	As your toddler's sleep needs evolve, it can be a bit of a juggling act, especially if you're managing other children, a full-time job and everything else on your plate. Toddlers need about 11 to 14 hours of sleep a day, including one or two naps. It can feel challenging to fit everything in – especially since not every toddler will be eager to nap when you might need that little break the most!
Preschoolers (3–5 years)	Preschoolers typically require about 10 to 13 hours of sleep each day, and you'll likely notice that daytime naps start to become less frequent. Some preschoolers might still enjoy a nap, while others begin to outgrow them, preferring to power through the day without one.

Your little one is eager to explore and assert their independence, and you need eyes in the back of your head. As they grow, their sleep starts to consolidate into longer night-time stretches, usually with one or two naps during the day. But with that comes some common challenges, like frequent awakenings and difficulties in self-soothing, as well as the transition into a 'big' bed and getting them to stay put all night.

Sleep disorders can pop up at any stage of life, and childhood is no exception. But before we dive into some of the more common issues, I want to take a moment to think about something that often gets overlooked: the roots of our own relationship with sleep.

Have you ever considered how much of what we believe and feel comes from our childhood? We soak up so much from our parents or caregivers, even things we might not consciously realise. I'll share a personal story – my mother tells a tale about how, as a child, I overheard my father say he didn't like onions. From that day on, I decided I didn't like onions either, and that's stuck with me even now. It makes you wonder, doesn't it – do I really not like onions, or is this just something I picked up from my dad?

Social learning

This is a process known as social learning.[14] When you were young, you were like a sponge, absorbing everything around you. You looked to your parents or caregivers to understand the world, including how to approach things like sleep.[15] If your parents were calm and reassuring about sleep, you likely internalised that way of being. But if they were anxious or stressed about it, you might have picked up on those feelings, too.[16]

Attachment theory plays into this as well. If you had a strong, secure bond with your parents or caregivers, you probably felt safe and were more likely to adopt their views and habits. But if there was a lot of stress or anxiety in your environment, your nervous system might have mirrored that, making it harder for you to relax and sleep well.

Children are incredibly perceptive – they pick up on both verbal and nonverbal cues. So, if your parent or caregiver often said things like, 'I never get enough sleep', or 'I dread bedtime', you might have started to feel the same way without even realising it. And it's not just the words – nonverbal cues like facial expressions and body language can convey just as much, if not more, than what's said out loud. I often think of the problem with the saying 'Don't do as I do, do as I say'. It highlights a common disconnect – it's an attempt to steer the child's behaviour through verbal instruction, even when actions contradict those instructions. However, children learn primarily through observation and imitation, not just through what we tell them. It's why the words we use around children matter so much – but our actions speak even louder.

We build mental frameworks based on our experiences. If bedtime was associated with anxiety or negativity, that might have become your script for what sleep is supposed to be like.[17] Emotions are another big piece of the puzzle. You learned how to handle your emotions by watching your parents or caregivers. If a parent or caregiver showed a lot of distress over sleeping poorly, you might have learned to associate sleep with stress and anxiety. It's like an emotional contagion – children often 'catch' the emotions their parents or caregivers are feeling.

I am absolutely not blaming parents or caregivers. This isn't about guilt; it's about understanding the circle of life and how we all naturally absorb and pass on beliefs, as well as offering insight into some of what might lie in the roots of your issue with sleep. In therapy, we often explore how the attitudes and beliefs we picked up as children stick with us into adulthood, and how they might not always serve us well. Becoming aware of these patterns gives us the chance to change them, for ourselves and for our children.

So, what can you do? Start by reflecting on your own childhood – what beliefs about sleep (or anything else) have you internalised that might not actually be yours? It's also important to be mindful of how you talk about sleep around your children. Using positive, empathetic language can make a big difference. Instead of saying, 'I never sleep well,' try framing it as, 'I'm working on getting better sleep.' It's about creating a healthy, positive outlook.

By being more aware of your words and actions, you can help your children develop healthier habits and attitudes. And remember, this isn't about striving for perfection – there's no such thing as a perfect parent or caregiver. But making small, intentional changes can have a big impact over time.

Primary-years children

Primary-years children (ages 6–12)	Primary-years children require 9–12 hours of sleep per night. Managing sleep disturbances involves encouraging a consistent sleep schedule, limiting screen time before bed and promoting a calm bedtime routine.[18]

As children move into the school years, you might notice that their sleep becomes a bit more settled compared to when they were younger. But that doesn't mean sleep disturbances disappear completely. With academic pressures, after-school activities and the lure of smartphones, sleep can still be a challenge. These factors might lead to trouble falling asleep, waking up during the night or even resisting bedtime altogether. Stress levels in the home can rapidly escalate when your child isn't going to bed when you want them to.

To support your child's sleep, there are a few things you can do that really make a difference. Encouraging plenty of natural light during the day – especially in the morning – can help regulate their sleep–wake cycle. Keeping a consistent sleep schedule, limiting screen time before bed and establishing a calming bedtime routine can also work wonders.

Children's sleep problems often have a lot to do with the stress they're experiencing from school and activities. It can be hard for them to wind down at night when their minds are still buzzing with the day's events.

I understand that many parents are turning to melatonin to help their children sleep, especially when they're struggling to fall asleep or their sleep schedules are out of sync. Melatonin can indeed be a helpful aid, but it's important to use it thoughtfully. There's still much we don't know about the long-term effects of melatonin in kids, and finding the right dose can be challenging. Since melatonin also plays a role in puberty, it's especially important to exercise caution when considering its use with teenagers.[19]

If you're considering melatonin – or any other medication or supplement – check in with a healthcare professional to see what else might be going on. There might be questions about neurodiversity, a circadian rhythm disorder, anxiety or something else.[20] Every child is different, and what works for one might not work for another. The key is to stay informed and make decisions that feel right for your family, without feeling pressured or overwhelmed.

At the end of the day, it's about finding what helps your child feel calm, safe and ready to rest, and that doesn't come in the form of a supplement. There's no one-size-fits-all approach to sleep, and you're the expert on what works best for your child.

Sleep disorders that appear in childhood

Sleep-onset association disorder

This behavioural insomnia is commonly seen in infants and young children who learn to fall asleep only under specific conditions, such as being rocked or fed or having to have a particular cuddly toy. Using sound or television as a sleep aid can be a double-edged sword: on the one hand, a consistent and soothing sound, like white noise or soft music, can help signal that it's time to sleep; on the other, relying on television or streaming is generally not recommended. The light and stimulation from the screen can interfere with the body's natural sleep rhythms and make it harder for a child to fall and stay asleep.

When these conditions are not present, they have difficulty falling asleep or returning to sleep during night-time awakenings. This can often be addressed with gradual sleep training and establishing consistent bedtime routines.

Sleepwalking and talking

NREM parasomnias are a group of sleep issues that include sleepwalking, night terrors and confusional arousals.[21] They usually happen during transitions between sleep stages, particularly during NREM sleep, leading to partial awakenings. When these things happen, it can be really unnerving as a parent, as your child might appear confused and may not respond to you.

They are relatively common, affecting about 20 per cent of children, and are considered a part of normal brain development. They tend to decrease with age, but a small percentage of individuals continue to experience these events into adulthood.[22]

Sleepwalking affects between 1 per cent and 15 per cent of the general population, and it is more common in children, particularly between the ages of four and eight.[23] If your child is a sleepwalker, make sure their environment is safe – it might be time to get the sleep gate out again to stop these nocturnal meanderings.

Nightmares and night terrors – two very different things

Memorable nightmares usually happen during the REM stage of sleep, which is predominantly in the second half of the night. They're those vivid, scary dreams that can wake up a child. Children (and adults) often wake up in tears, scared of the monster in their dream. They will be fully awake and able to tell you all about it. As a parent you need to comfort them; reassure them that it was just a dream and not real, and stay with them until they feel safe. You don't necessarily need to be there until they fall asleep again, as this can create a problematic loop in future. Maybe read a soothing book, give them their favourite stuffed animal and leave a red night light on for them to fall asleep again.

It is believed that one of the reasons nightmares happen is that the brain is trying to deal with unresolved issues or fears and is a sign of a healthy mind – however distressing.[24] This idea comes from psychological theories about why we dream. One well-known theory is called the continuity hypothesis, which suggests that our dreams mirror our waking thoughts, worries and experiences.[25] According to this theory, there's a connection between what we go through during the day and what we dream about at night. Our dreams, including nightmares, often reflect our daily concerns and emotions. Research has shown that stressful or traumatic experiences can make nightmares more frequent, supporting the idea that nightmares are the brain's way of processing these events.

Night terrors are different. As we saw in Chapter One, they usually happen during the first third of the night, during deep NREM sleep. When your child has one, they might sit up suddenly, scream or thrash around, looking terrified. But here's the thing – they are not fully awake and won't respond to you. In the morning, they won't remember it at all. It can be hard to deal with and deeply upsetting as your child may be screaming the house down, deeply distressed. The best thing to do is to stay calm. Trying to wake them doesn't help and can make things worse. Make sure they are safe, gently guide them back to bed if they get up and wait it out. Most of the time, it's over in a few minutes and they go back to sleep.

Just remember, both are common. Most children outgrow them as they get older, but if they're happening a lot or really affecting your daily life, it might be good to talk to a paediatrician or a sleep specialist.

No matter your age, there are steps you can take to reduce the likelihood of experiencing nightmares or night terrors. One of the most effective strategies is maintaining a consistent bedtime routine. Over-tiredness and missing your natural sleep window can be triggers for these episodes. Establishing a calming bedtime routine can make a significant difference – try incorporating a warm bath, reading a book or dimming the lights before bed to help your body unwind.

It's also worth revisiting the technique mentioned above on page 31 – Justin Havens's method for transforming nightmares. If you find yourself frequently plagued by disturbing dreams, Havens's approach of reimagining the nightmare's ending in a positive way can be incredibly effective. By practising this technique, you can take control of your dreams and reduce the impact of nightmares on your sleep.

Finally, be mindful of what you expose yourself to before bed. Avoid watching scary movies or engaging with stressful content late at night, as these can influence your sleep and increase the chances of experiencing nightmares or night terrors. By creating a peaceful sleep environment and sticking to a soothing routine, along with using techniques like Havens's, you can help reduce these unsettling sleep disturbances at any age.

Obstructive sleep apnea (OSA)

When we think of sleep apnea, we usually picture it as an adult issue, but it's important to recognise that children can experience it too. In kids, obstructive sleep apnea (OSA) is often due to enlarged tonsils or adenoids. You might notice symptoms like snoring, pauses in breathing, or restless sleep. If this sounds familiar, it's worth getting it checked out. Sometimes the solution might be surgery to remove the tonsils and adenoids, or the use of continuous positive airway pressure (CPAP) therapy. There's also been a rise in sleep apnea among children, and unfortunately, obesity is a significant contributing factor.[26] Being aware of these possibilities means you can take early action.

Teenagers and young adults

Teenagers (ages 13–18)	Significant biological and social changes can impact sleep patterns. Teenagers need about 8–10 hours of sleep each night, but many don't get enough because of early school start times, social activities and the increased use of electronic devices.
Young adults (ages 18–25)	Remember that many teenagers and young adults are night owls squeezed into a social timeframe at odds with their biological clock.

Teenagers and sleep. It's such a challenging time, isn't it? The teenage years bring about so many biological and social changes, and these really do impact sleep patterns. Teenagers typically need about eight to ten hours of sleep each night, but getting enough sleep is often easier said than done. Early school starts, social activities and all those electronic devices – they really don't help, do they?

Remember the section earlier in the book where I stress the importance of being sleepy to be able to go to sleep? If your teenager stays up late and struggles to get up in the morning, you might be frustrated, but it's not just them being difficult. They might not be sleepy at the time needed for them to go to bed to get the sleep that they need. There's a biological reason for it. During puberty, it's normal for the body's internal clock to shift, causing teenagers to naturally want to go to bed later and wake up later. This shift is part of typical adolescent development and is often referred to as a delayed sleep phase. However, delayed sleep phase disorder (DSPD) is more extreme. DSPD occurs when this shift becomes so pronounced that it significantly interferes with daily life, making it very difficult for them to fall asleep and wake up at socially acceptable times, even when they try. While many teens experience a later sleep preference, DSPD affects about 7 to 16 per cent of them,[27] causing chronic sleep disruption that impacts school, work and social responsibilities.

Puberty itself ends when their bones stop growing – usually around age 16 for girls and 17 and a half for boys. But adolescence, with all its physical, psychological, social and mental changes, stretches a bit longer, ending around age 19. During this time, they have this seemingly endless ability to stay up late and sleep in. Between the ages of 20 and 26, though, their internal clock starts to shift earlier again. By the time they're 55, they'll naturally wake up at around the same time they did when they were 10.[28]

This connection between the biological clock and the end of puberty is so strong that some researchers believe this 'peak lateness' could even be a biological marker signalling the end of puberty. And for some, this tendency to stay up late can extend into their mid-20s as their brain continues to mature. So, if your teenager, or even your young adult child, has always struggled with sleep, it's important to understand that it's not just a lack of discipline. Their biological clock might still be in the process of adjusting and they might be biological night owls.

As they transition into a 9-to-5 world, this natural inclination to stay up late can make things even tougher. Understanding these shifts in sleep patterns matters, so that you appreciate how forcing them into a routine that doesn't fit their biology causes problems. It's about helping them – and you – navigate this phase with more understanding and compassion. Sometimes just recognising that there's a biological reason behind your sleep patterns can make all the difference. If this is happening in your home, seek help as there are ways to treat it.

Narcolepsy and cataplexy

Narcolepsy, though rare, usually appears during adolescence or young adulthood. It's linked to a genetic marker that makes a person more vulnerable to an autoimmune response, which can attack specific neurons in the brain that help regulate wakefulness. Environmental triggers, like infections or certain vaccines, can set off this response, leading to symptoms such as vivid dreams, sleep paralysis, sudden 'sleep attacks' and even hallucinations.[29]

Some people with narcolepsy also experience cataplexy, which is a sudden loss of muscle control triggered by strong emotions like laughter, surprise or frustration. Cataplexy can range from mild – such as drooping eyelids or a slack jaw – to more dramatic episodes where a person may briefly collapse while fully aware. People with narcolepsy often experience very vivid dreams and can even have lucid dreams, where they're aware they're dreaming. These unique symptoms can make living with someone with narcolepsy a bit challenging, but understanding them is a big step towards finding the right ways to manage and cope.

Despite memes and comedy sketches suggesting otherwise, narcolepsy is no joke; it can be a significant disability, profoundly impacting daily life. Approximately 1 in 2,500 people in the UK are affected, meaning around 30,000 people have it, though many remain undiagnosed. It can severely disrupt education, employment, driving, relationships and emotional health. While there is no cure, effective medications and strategies can help manage symptoms, enabling those with narcolepsy to lead full lives.[30]

Historically, narcolepsy was misunderstood and once thought to be linked to encephalitis lethargica, a post-World War I condition. Encephalitis lethargica, also known as 'sleepy sickness', peaked between 1916 and 1927.[31] The disease presented with symptoms such as high fever, headache, lethargy and double vision – often progressing to neurological complications like parkinsonism and catatonia. The exact cause of encephalitis lethargica remains unknown, though some hypotheses suggest it was triggered by an autoimmune response to the influenza virus.

A significant breakthrough came from studying dogs with a genetic form of narcolepsy.[32] This led Professor Emmanuel Mignot at Stanford University and Masashi Yanagisawa at the University of Tsukuba to discover that those with the condition have low levels of hypocretin (orexin), a neuropeptide regulating wakefulness and appetite. They were awarded the prestigious 2023 Breakthrough Prize in Life Sciences for their significant contributions to understanding narcolepsy, which underscores the impact of their discovery on the field of sleep disorders and neurodegenerative disease research.

Understanding and managing narcolepsy and cataplexy can significantly improve quality of life. If you suspect that you or someone you know has narcolepsy, seek medical advice for proper diagnosis and treatment.

Adulthood, with its many stages, trials and tribulations

In this section, we'll dip into the different stages of adulthood – not every twist and turn, but enough to explore how these phases affect your relationship with sleep, rest and wellbeing.

The emerging years (18–29)

- Your 20s are a decade of self-discovery, where you're figuring out what you want from life and the direction you're heading – both personally and professionally. But with this freedom also comes a fair share of instability and unpredictability.
- Though it may not seem pressing now, the habits formed during these years – how you manage stress, how much sleep you get, how you balance work and fun – shape how you handle challenges down the road. It's a time for exploration, but also for laying the groundwork for long-term stability.

Common sleep issues
- **Sleep deprivation:** With a social life that often stretches into the early morning hours and the demands of your new career or studies, it's easy to sacrifice sleep. You might find yourself prioritising fun or work over rest, thinking you can catch up later, but the truth is, it adds up and can leave you feeling drained.
- **Irregular sleep patterns:** Your routine is likely changing a lot – different work shifts, spontaneous nights out or pulling all-nighters for exams. These frequent changes can really mess with your sleep cycle, making it hard to maintain a regular sleep schedule.
- **Insomnia:** While insomnia can happen at any age, the excitement and anxiety that come with navigating new responsibilities can

sometimes keep you up at night. It's a common issue when you're dealing with so much change and uncertainty.

- **Teenage biological clock:** As we have seen previously as you move through your early to mid-20s, your body might still be running on a bit of a teenage biological clock. During adolescence, your internal clock naturally shifts to a later schedule, making it tough to fall asleep early and wake up early. This shift can stick around, which might make you more inclined to stay up late and sleep in. But when you're trying to adapt to the typical 9-to-5 schedule of adult life, this can create a real challenge, contributing to sleep deprivation and those irregular sleep patterns we just talked about.

Understanding these common sleep issues can help you be more aware of what's going on with your body and mind. You're navigating a lot during these years, and it's perfectly normal to experience some sleep disruptions. The important thing is to recognise them and think about how you might make small adjustments to improve your sleep and overall wellbeing.

Circadian rhythm sleep–wake disorders

Let's talk about circadian rhythm sleep–wake disorders (CRSWD). These are conditions where your natural sleep–wake cycle gets disrupted, either because your internal body clock is malfunctioning or because it's out of sync with the external world. This can happen at any age, and it can really affect how you function day-to-day, as well as interfering with your mental wellbeing.

CRSWDs are considered to have a strong neurological component. These disorders involve disruptions to the body's internal clock, which is regulated by the brain. The primary neurological structure responsible for regulating circadian rhythms is the suprachiasmatic nucleus (SCN), a tiny region of the hypothalamus in the brain. The SCN acts as the body's 'master clock', coordinating the timing of various physiological processes, including sleep–wake cycles, hormone release and body temperature.

When the SCN or other parts of the brain that regulate sleep and wakefulness are impaired – whether due to injury, disease or other factors – circadian rhythms can become misaligned, leading to CRSWDs. These disruptions can manifest as difficulties in falling asleep, waking up too early, or sleeping at irregular times that don't align with societal norms or environmental cues.

In addition to neurological underpinnings, CRSWDs can also be influenced by genetic factors, lifestyle choices and environmental factors, such as exposure to light and work schedules. While the exact mechanisms of CRSWDs are complex and multifactorial, their basis in the brain's regulation of time-sensitive processes means they are often classified and treated within the context of neurological and sleep medicine.

There are different types of CRSWD to consider:
- **Delayed sleep–wake phase disorder**: where you struggle to fall asleep until very late at night.
- **Advanced sleep–wake phase disorder**: which causes you to wake up unusually early.
- **Non-24-hour sleep–wake rhythm disorder**: where your sleep times gradually shift, making it hard to stick to a regular schedule.
- **Irregular sleep–wake rhythm disorder**: which is marked by inconsistent sleep episodes scattered throughout the day.

These disorders can have a significant impact not only on you but on those around you. A lot of people I've worked with share how socially, these disorders can be really isolating, especially if they interfere with your ability to work or maintain relationships. You are constantly out of step with the world. It's no wonder this can lead to feelings of depression.

Unfortunately, sleep disorders like these aren't always well understood, and people can sometimes unfairly blame you, as if it's something you should be able to control easily. But the truth is, these are complex issues, and they require understanding and appropriate treatment to help you manage them effectively.

Shift work sleep disorder (SWSD)
While some level of fatigue is normal for anyone working irregular hours, shift work sleep disorder (SWSD) happens when the misalignment between an individual's internal clock and their work schedule leads to persistent and significant problems with sleep. Those with

SWSD experience chronic excessive sleepiness or insomnia, which interferes with daily functioning and overall wellbeing. If these symptoms persist despite attempts to adjust, SWSD may be present.

Seasonal mood and behaviour (seasonal rhythms)

You might have noticed how your mood shifts with the changing seasons. These fluctuations are natural and closely tied to the circadian rhythm. For many people, these seasonal mood changes are mild – a slight dip in energy during the winter or a burst of liveliness as spring arrives. However, for some, the shifts are more intense. You might have heard of seasonal affective disorder (SAD), a type of depression that typically occurs during the darker months. It's not just feeling a bit down; it involves a significant drop in mood and energy that can deeply affect daily life. If you're experiencing these symptoms, seeking support and exploring treatment options is important.

The establishing years (30–39)

By the time you reach your 30s, you might find yourself in the midst of building a career, possibly starting a family and putting down roots. This decade often brings a more structured routine, but it also comes with increased responsibilities. The demands on your time and energy can be significant, leading to a juggling act that often leaves you feeling exhausted.

Common sleep issues
- **Work-related stress:** the pressures of advancing in your career can lead to stress, affecting the ability to wind down.
- **Parental sleep deprivation:** for those with young children, disrupted nights become common as you navigate the sleeplessness that comes with parenting.
- **Restless legs syndrome (RLS):** this disorder involves an irresistible urge to move the legs, typically occurring in the evening or night-time. RLS can begin in adolescence and is associated with discomfort or tingling sensations in the legs. Also known as Willis–Ekbom disease, it's far more than just a minor annoyance – it can be utterly debilitating for those who live with

it. Some people experience the same uncomfortable sensations – such as tingling, creeping, or pulling – in other parts of the body, like the arms, torso and even the face. It often appears during pregnancy, may be linked to iron deficiency, and treatment can include iron supplements and lifestyle changes.

- **Periodic limb movement disorder (PLMD):** if you sleep alone, you might not know you have this. Characterised by repetitive limb movements during sleep, PLMD can disrupt sleep and lead to daytime fatigue. It is more common in adults and can be treated with medications that reduce limb movements or improve sleep quality.

The settling years (40–49)

This decade often brings a sense of stability and purpose, but it also comes with heightened responsibilities. Balancing work, family and personal goals can feel like a constant juggling act, with more demands on your time and energy than ever. Physically, you might notice that your body doesn't bounce back as quickly as it once did, or that fatigue lingers longer. Some people are also balancing the needs of ageing parents alongside raising children, adding another layer of emotional and logistical strain.

Common sleep issues
- **Hormonal changes:** for women, peri-menopause can bring hot flushes and night sweats, disrupting sleep.
- **Chronic stress:** ongoing career and family responsibilities can continue to impact sleep quality.
- **Early signs of chronic conditions:** issues like hypertension or arthritis can begin to interfere with restful sleep.
- **Sleep apnea:** this is a period when sleep apnea can become more apparent, particularly if lifestyle changes have led to weight gain.

The reflective years (50–59)

Reaching your 50s it's natural to start looking back over your life, particularly as your children begin to leave the nest and the prospect of retirement draws nearer. But in the middle of that you may well still be going at a million miles an hour. This stage of life can bring a mix of emotions – there's often a sense of newfound freedom, but it can also be accompanied by the challenges of ageing, such as more fragmented sleep or the cumulative effects of stress and poor sleep over the years. It's important to acknowledge these changes and find ways to navigate them with care and self-compassion.

Common sleep issues

- **Menopausal symptoms:** continued hormonal fluctuations can cause sleep disturbances for women.
- **Sleep maintenance insomnia:** difficulty staying asleep becomes more common, often due to health issues or the natural ageing process.
- **Nocturia:** frequent urination at night, or nocturia, is common in older adults and can significantly disrupt sleep. Causes include enlarged prostate in men, urinary tract infections and diabetes. Treatment involves managing the underlying condition, reducing fluid intake before bed and, sometimes, medication.

REM sleep behaviour disorder

During REM sleep, your body naturally experiences temporary paralysis to prevent you from acting out your dreams, while your breathing and heart rate continue as normal. In rare cases, if this paralysis doesn't occur, it could be due to a condition called REM sleep behaviour disorder (RBD). People with RBD might physically act out their dreams, which can sometimes lead to minor injuries for themselves or their bed partner. Research shows that 30–60 per cent of people with RBD have accidentally hurt themselves, while 30–50 per cent have injured their bed partner. These injuries can range from small bruises to more serious cuts.[33] RBD is relatively uncommon, affecting approximately 0.5 per cent to 1 per cent of the general population. It's more frequently observed in older adults, particularly men over the age of 50. While the condition is rare, it's important to note that its prevalence can increase in individuals with certain neurodegenerative conditions like Parkinson's disease, where it might be seen in up to 25–50 per cent of cases.[34]

So, while RBD is something to be aware of, especially if you or someone you know shows symptoms, it's not something most people will experience. If there are concerns, it's always best to consult with a healthcare provider to discuss any potential symptoms and receive appropriate guidance.

The wisdom years (60–79)

As we move into our 60s and 70s, life often begins to slow down, giving us more time for rest and reflection. However, sleep disturbances become increasingly common at this stage, affecting between 39 and 75 per cent of this group.[35] These disturbances manifest as fatigue, emotional distress, anxiety, difficulty concentrating, memory issues, daytime dysfunction and an increased risk of falls, collectively diminishing overall health and quality of life.[36]

One major transition during this period is retirement. For many, this shift brings a mix of emotions – there's excitement and a sense of liberation, but also fear and anxiety – due to your financial situation retirement might still be a long way off. After decades of routine, stepping into retirement can feel like a leap of faith. While it may offer relief from the stresses of work and more free time, it can also lead to deep questions about your identity and sense of self. The change in routine, for instance, can disrupt your sleep patterns, and a decrease in physical and social activities – both of which tie in to healthy sleep – can further exacerbate the issue.[37] Moreover, the psychological adjustment to retirement shouldn't be underestimated. Finding a new sense of purpose, managing any financial concerns and redefining your role in society can all contribute to sleep challenges. Many people, although financially prepared for retirement, find themselves mentally unprepared for the profound changes it brings. This transition can involve a partial disruption of identity, indecision, a loss of self-confidence, feelings of emptiness and a search for meaningful engagement in the community.[38]

This stage of life also brings with it the increased risk of losing loved ones and friends. Grief becomes a more frequent companion, and it's essential to seek support when dealing with such losses. Navigating the intersection of ageing and retirement requires creating a new structure for your life, addressing anxiety about mortality, maintaining important social relationships and grappling with evolving questions of self-identity. It's a time of great change, and it's OK to seek help as you move through these transitions.

David sits on the edge of the chair, his fingers drumming a nervous rhythm on the armrest. 'How have you been?' I ask, though the answer is already apparent in his tense posture. The past few months have weighed heavily on him – work projects reaching a crescendo, family tensions simmering just below the surface. But what truly gnaws at him is the looming shadow of retirement. 'I don't feel my age. I'm still sharp, still capable. But it's like the world is telling me it's time to step aside, to fade out, just because I've hit some arbitrary number. It feels like I'm being handed a death sentence I'm not ready for.'

David has always been deeply connected to his work; we've spoken many times about how it anchors him, gives him purpose. I ask him how this growing pressure to retire has been affecting him. He leans back, pressing his fingers to his temples as if trying to knead away the tension. 'It's been relentless,' he admits. 'The insomnia's been a constant. Years now, waking up at 3 a.m., my mind buzzing with all the things I've got to do. Time feels like it's running out. It's exhausting.'

Our work together began with his insomnia, but it quickly became clear that his sleepless nights were just the tip of a much larger iceberg. The prospect of change – of stepping away from the life he's built – terrifies him. It's a fear I've seen many times: the paradox of needing to slow down but being utterly resistant to it. We've discussed the usual remedies – breathing exercises, mindfulness, cutting back on caffeine – but David finds these suggestions insubstantial. His mind is a high-speed train, and there's no off switch.

This relentless pace has been his way of life for so long. It's not just the work itself, but what it represents – a pillar of his identity. The thought of retirement feels like being put out to pasture, a forced obsolescence after years of dedicated toil. It's not simply about leaving work behind; it's about losing a part of himself.

Retirement doesn't have to mean an end to your contributions or your sense of purpose. It could be an opportunity to refocus your energy on things you've always wanted to do but never had the time for. Have you thought about what those might be?

The 60s, the 70s – these years demand a redefinition of purpose. The roles that once defined you begin to shift or fall away, and what's left can feel unsettling, even frightening. But within that void lies opportunity – a chance to explore new avenues, to rekindle relationships, to find joy in activities that perhaps were neglected. Meaningful engagement isn't just a balm for the restless mind. A life with purpose tends to lead to better sleep, because a fulfilled mind is less likely to wrestle with itself in the dead of night.

It's also important to dispel the myth that poor sleep is an inevitable part of ageing. It's true that as we age, sleep patterns change – more frequent awakenings, less deep sleep, more time spent in lighter stages of sleep.[39] Ageing is associated with decreased REM sleep, increased sleep fragmentation, shorter total sleep duration and lower sleep efficiency.[40] The coveted sleep of youth may no longer be within reach, and part of our work together is reconciling with that reality. Expectations need adjustment, not just habits.

So, what do we do? We prioritise and protect sleep. Consistent wake times, a restful environment, stress management – these are relevant at every stage of life. Embracing these practices won't turn back the clock, but they can help you age with a sense of wellbeing and grace, giving you the tools to navigate the inevitable changes that come with growing older.

Common sleep issues

- **Chronic pain:** conditions such as arthritis or back pain can significantly disrupt sleep.
- **Increased risk of sleep apnea:** often requiring medical intervention.
- **Advanced sleep phase disorder (ASPD):** typically seen in older adults, ASPD involves an early evening sleep onset and early morning awakening. This disorder is related to changes in the circadian rhythm that occur with ageing. Treatment may include light therapy in the evening and melatonin supplements.

- **Insomnia related to chronic conditions:** in older adults, insomnia can often be secondary to chronic health conditions such as arthritis, heart disease or depression. Treating the underlying condition and incorporating better sleep practices can help improve sleep.

The golden years (80 and beyond): embracing rest and reflection

As we move into our 80s and beyond, life naturally slows down, allowing for a more reflective and introspective pace. This period, often called the 'golden years', can indeed be a time of profound personal growth and deepened connections with others. However, it also comes with its own set of challenges. Sleep can become even more fragmented and elusive, and any health issues you may have encountered in your 60s and 70s can continue or become more pronounced.

In these later years, sleep disturbances are unfortunately very common. Many older adults find it difficult to stay asleep throughout the night, often waking up multiple times or finding themselves awake in the early hours of the morning.[41] This can lead to symptoms such as fatigue, confusion and mood swings, which can significantly affect your daily functioning and overall wellbeing.[42] Additionally, neurological conditions like dementia and Parkinson's disease, which are more prevalent in this age group, can severely impact your sleep patterns and those around you.[43]

Sundowning syndrome

Alzheimer's disease can severely disrupt sleep, leaving both the individual and their caregiver feeling constantly exhausted. As the disease progresses, it becomes harder for the brain to regulate the sleep–wake cycle, which can lead to trouble falling asleep, frequent awakenings, and increased restlessness or confusion at night – a pattern often called 'sundowning'.[44] These sleep challenges not only make it harder to get restful sleep but also add to the cognitive and emotional difficulties of the disease, making each day feel a little more challenging for everyone involved.

For caregivers, this relentless disruption of sleep is incredibly hard. The constant vigilance required to ensure their loved one's safety during the night means that they, too, suffer from chronic sleep deprivation. Over time, the physical and emotional toll of these sleepless nights can become overwhelming, making the decision to consider residential care a painful, yet often necessary, step.

Tips for managing sundowning[45]

- Use distraction techniques: go into a different room, make the person a drink, have a snack, turn some music on or go out for a walk.
- If possible, regular physical activity, even gentle exercises like walking or stretching, can promote better sleep.[46]
- Ask them what the matter is. Listen carefully to their response and if possible, see if you can deal with the reason for their distress.
- Talk in a slow, soothing way.
- Speak in short sentences and give simple instructions to try to avoid confusion.
- Hold the person's hand or sit close to them and stroke their arm.

Summary

Sleep is a universal yet deeply personal experience, shaped by our biology, life stage and environment. From the sleepless nights of new parenthood to the disrupted rhythms of shift work, to the challenges of ageing, each phase of life brings unique hurdles and needs. Sleep issues are rarely isolated – they are the result of intricate interactions between the body, mind and world around us.

This chapter is not about self-diagnosing or quick fixes but about understanding sleep disorders in their full context. By tuning in to your patterns, documenting your experiences and seeking support when needed, you can better advocate for yourself and work towards restful, restorative sleep. Whether it's recognising the impact of societal pressures, exploring underlying psychological connections or addressing biological factors like circadian rhythms, the key is awareness. Sleep is not just a necessity – it's a reflection of how we live.

Final thoughts from me

As a psychotherapist, I witness first-hand the profound impact that sleep – or the lack of it – has on every facet of our lives. Sleep is often seen as a passive state, but it is anything but. It reflects how we live, relate to ourselves and interact with others. Over time, I've come to realise that sleep is not merely the final chapter of our day. It's a mirror that reflects how we spend our waking hours. It's easy to see sleep as something elusive, but perhaps the real elusiveness lies in the balance we struggle to find between productivity and rest, between control and surrender.

My ongoing inquiry centres on this connection: how our existence – our sense of self, our interactions with the world and the demands placed upon us – directly influences how we rest. When we haven't slept well, who are we? Our very personality shifts with the quality of our sleep. This realisation was part of what drew me to specialise in sleep. As a psychotherapist, I began to see the profound impact that sleep – or the lack of it – has on our emotional lives, our resilience, our ability to engage with the work of therapy. I started to wonder: what are we doing in therapy if either the client, or even the therapist, has an undiagnosed sleep issue? How effective can we be in exploring the layers of the psyche when one of us is running on empty? And so, sleep became my focus. Through the biopsychosocial lens, we can see that sleep is not just a biological need – it's a process influenced by how we live, how we think and how we connect with those around us.

From infancy to old age, sleep is woven into the fabric of our being, evolving with us. Hormonal changes throughout life – during puberty, pregnancy and menopause – further reveal the deep biological ties to sleep.

Sleep disturbances, particularly those linked to psychological factors, illustrate how interconnected we are with our internal and external worlds. Anxiety, depression, and stress are not only consequences of poor sleep but also contributors. Through psychotherapy, cognitive behavioural therapy for insomnia (CBT-I) and other psychological interventions, I've seen how addressing these underlying issues can dramatically improve one's quality of life. And when we look at chronic conditions like sleep apnea, narcolepsy or cataplexy, the emotional toll cannot be ignored. Psychotherapy becomes not just a tool for symptom management but a lifeline for coping with the psychological strain these conditions bring.

Our relationships and environments deeply influence our sleep. The isolation experienced by many older adults further underscores how intertwined sleep and social connection are. Sleep is not just an individual issue, but a communal one, requiring societal structures that promote and prioritise rest.

We live in a world that often works against the quiet, restorative space that sleep requires. The fast-paced demands of modern life, with its focus on productivity and constant connectivity, leave little room for reflection, stillness or genuine rest. Environmental factors, including the quality of the air we breathe and the spaces we inhabit, also impact our ability to recharge. The foods we consume – often loaded with chemicals, sugar and empty calories – can disrupt our bodies' natural rhythms, contributing to insomnia, anxiety and conditions like sleep apnea.

The societal pressures placed upon us – work schedules, economic challenges and social expectations – make restful sleep seem like a luxury rather than the fundamental necessity it is. From new parents struggling without sufficient support to sleep-deprived adolescents buckling under academic pressures, to adults juggling the unrelenting demands of work, caregiving and financial stress, our nights are consumed by the pressures of our days. Even older adults, often isolated or under-supported, feel the effects of a society that values productivity over presence. In this landscape, good sleep isn't just hard to come by – it's eroded by the very systems that should support it.

But sleep is more than a biological need; it is a vital process, a reflection of how we live, connect and find meaning in a world that often leaves little room for introspection. The keys to peaceful sleep lie in the quiet moments we carve out, the connections we nourish and the anxieties we untangle.

As I continue my ongoing inquiry into sleep, I'm reminded time and again that sleep disturbances are often not individual failures but symptoms of a life out of sync. How we spend our days – the stress, the rushing, the relentless demands – determines how we spend our nights. When we are deprived of calm and space during the day, our nights reflect that turbulence. The world we've created – with its nonstop distractions, environmental challenges and disconnection from nature – creates the perfect conditions for sleeplessness.

When we rest, we begin to rise.

Sleep responds to care, attention and presence. And just as the forces around us shape our sleep, so too can it be reclaimed by the choices we make – how we choose to live our days, how we care for our bodies and minds, and how we protect the spaces that nurture rest.

This isn't just an individual journey; it's a collective one. As a society, we must foster environments that value wellbeing and promote the conditions necessary for rest. We need communities that support each other and systems that recognise rest as a fundamental human need, not a luxury. Good sleep is not a personal indulgence – it's a societal necessity.

Every time you choose rest – every time you embrace stillness or let go of the constant push to do more – you resist the pressures that tell you exhaustion is inevitable. You step towards a fuller, more meaningful existence.

Sleep becomes not just a biological need but a quiet revolution. So, in your pursuit of rest, remember this: how you spend your days is how you spend your nights. To sleep well is to live well. And as we let go each night, we wake up not only to a more rested body but to a life filled with more meaning – and a world that supports our need for rest.

Acknowledgements

Confidentiality is not just a professional standard; it's the bedrock of trust between therapist and client. As a psychotherapist, I've woven real-life struggles into this narrative, but none of them are lifted from our private exchanges. Your story is safe with me. If, by chance, you see yourself reflected in these words, it's because the pain of sleepless nights is so deeply human, so shared. The dance with disordered sleep is universal, with common threads running through each story of restless tossing, weary mornings and longing for peace.

Writing this book has been a humbling process. I've ventured far beyond the familiar contours of my psychotherapy practice, engaging with experts across fields who've offered their insights into sleep, biology and the mind. Their knowledge has filled in the gaps where my curiosity stretches beyond my expertise.

Thank you to those who have read drafts of these chapters; you have kept me grounded, making sure that what you read here is not only meaningful but accurate. Any mistakes are mine.

There are so many others who, while not my clients, have shared their stories with me, shaping and inspiring the words in this book and continuing to teach me what it means to be human. As a psychotherapist who has chosen to specialise in sleep, I often grapple with the delicate balance of honouring my clients' experiences while translating the complexities of sleep into something accessible and meaningful.

I apologise in advance for anything I may have misunderstood or not captured fully – I am always acutely aware of the immense responsibility of being a psychotherapist. It is a role I hold with care, humility, and the constant desire to learn and grow.

To my clients: it is a privilege to work with you. Thank you for trusting me with your stories and allowing me to walk alongside you on your journeys. Your courage, resilience and openness have taught me lessons that go far beyond therapy – lessons about life, humanity and the strength it takes to show up as your true self. You are, without question, my greatest teachers, and I am endlessly grateful for all you have shared with me.

The list of people who have helped me along the way is long, and I want to extend my heartfelt thanks to each and everyone of you.

To my agent, Jane Graham-Maw, a curious series of events brought us together, and I couldn't be more thankful. Your unwavering support and patience, along with that of Amy O'Shea, have meant so much to me. Thank you for believing in this book and guiding me through the process.

To Cyan Turan – thank you for believing in my idea and returning at just the right moment! To Julia Pollacco and the incredible team at Thorsons and HarperCollins, I'm deeply grateful to all of you.

To Dr Petra Hawker, Professor Guy Leschziner, Professor Russell Foster, Professor Adrian Williams, Professor Allison Harvey, Dr David O'Regan, Joanna Hogan, Peter Mansbach PhD, Charlie Morley, Dr Justin Havens, Dr Stephen Porges, Justin Sunseri, Ulysse Dormy from Atrim Ltd, Rebecca Algie from Lumie, Simon Chester, Rebecca Saul, David Yaffey, Susan Jordan, Janet Croft, Anna Menzies and Iona Menzies – thank you for your contributions, wisdom and support. Your insights have profoundly shaped my thinking and this book.

To the many others who, though not my clients, have shared your stories with me: your honesty and vulnerability have been a source of deep inspiration. Your experiences have informed these pages in ways you may not even realise. Thank you.

To Colin Cooper, thank you for your editing expertise and incredible patience. Your steady guidance has made this book so much better than it would have been otherwise.

Finally, to my family: the biggest thanks of all. You have endured the ups and downs of this book-writing journey with so much grace.

Tim and Harry, you are my sun, moon and stars. Your love, your humour and your endless patience have been my lifeline. This book has been a wild ride of excitement and despair, yet you have stood by me through it all. Thank you for grounding me, keeping me going and reminding me that I am never alone.

Dr Peter Gilliver and Dr Robin Darwall-Smith, your wisdom and kindness have been invaluable. I truly don't know how I would have managed without you. Thank you for being my guides when I felt lost.

And to Bella and Luna, my ever-faithful companions: dogs really do hold the secret to life, don't they? I once saw someone share how, after years of searching for meaning, they found themselves staring at the word 'dog' on a bowl and realised it was 'God' spelled backwards. It made perfect sense. You remind me every day of the power of presence, the beauty of unconditional love and the gift of living fully in the moment. Thank you for being my teachers and my joy.

This book is for all of you. Thank you.

Appendix

This section gathers additional information, resources and practical tips that didn't quite fit into the main chapters but might still be useful to you. Think of it as a toolkit – extra details and suggestions to support you on your journey to better sleep and wellbeing.

How much sleep do I need?

The US National Sleep Foundation suggests that most adults aim for seven to nine hours of sleep per night. If you're curious, their detailed sleep duration recommendations can be found here: https://www.thensf.org/how-many-hours-of-sleep-do-you-really-need/.

But here's the thing: sleep is personal. While these numbers provide a useful guideline, what works for one person may not work for another. Some people feel refreshed with seven hours, while others thrive closer to nine. That said, consistently getting less than six hours can start to take a toll, increasing your risk of poor focus, weakened immunity, and even long-term health issues like heart disease and diabetes.

The key is to pay attention to your body. If you're often tired, struggling to focus or not performing at your best, it could be a sign that you need more sleep. Try aiming for at least six hours as a baseline, but know that adding even an extra hour or two to your routine can make a noticeable difference in how you feel day-to-day. Sleep isn't about hitting a perfect number – it's about finding what helps you feel rested and ready to take on the day.

Who should and shouldn't do sleep restriction therapy?

Sleep restriction therapy (SRT) is a behavioural treatment for insomnia that involves limiting the time spent in bed to match the actual amount of sleep a person is getting, gradually increasing it as sleep improves. People may experience increased daytime sleepiness in the first one or two weeks of treatment. There are certain groups of people for whom SRT might not be suitable:

- **Individuals with bipolar disorder:** Sleep deprivation can trigger manic episodes in people with bipolar disorder, making SRT potentially harmful.[1]
- **People with epilepsy:** Sleep deprivation can increase the risk of seizures, so individuals with epilepsy might not be suitable candidates for SRT.[2]
- **Those with severe obstructive sleep apnea (OSA):** While SRT is used as part of CBT-I with those who have co-morbid insomnia and sleep apnea (COMISA), those with severe obstructive sleep apnea (OSA), managing both conditions together through a tailored approach is essential and requires professional guidance.
- **People with certain medical conditions:** Conditions that require longer sleep durations for recovery, such as recent surgery, chronic pain or severe depression, might make SRT unsuitable.
- **Shift workers:** Individuals with irregular sleep schedules due to shift work may find SRT challenging to implement effectively.
- **Severe anxiety disorders:** SRT can initially increase sleep anxiety, so those with severe anxiety may need alternative treatments or a combination of therapies.

How to explore ACE (adverse childhood experiences)

Many websites offer a version of the ACE questionnaire for free, but if you're interested in understanding your ACE score within a broader context, it's a good idea to talk to a professional such as a therapist, counsellor or healthcare provider. They can include the test as part of a more comprehensive mental health evaluation and interpret the results in a way that makes sense for your specific situation. They can also provide guidance on how childhood experiences may be influencing your health and wellbeing today, and offer steps for healing and resilience.

Keep in mind:

- **Your ACE score is just a starting point:** While it's useful in understanding how early experiences may have shaped your health and behaviour, it's not the sole determinant of your future. Many factors, including resilience, support systems and therapy, play a role in overcoming ACEs.
- **Look for trauma-informed professionals:** If you're exploring your ACE score with the help of a therapist, try to find one who has experience with trauma and childhood adversity. They can help you process the results in a safe and supportive way.

How to access CBT-I in the UK

If you're struggling with insomnia and are interested in trying cognitive behavioural therapy for insomnia (CBT-I), there are several ways you can access it here in the UK. As a psychotherapist, I often integrate CBT-I into my work (and throughout this book). Here's how you can access it:

Through the NHS:

- **GP referral:** Your first step should be talking to your GP. They can refer you to a sleep specialist or a psychologist who offers CBT-I. This may involve one-on-one sessions, group therapy or online programmes.
- **IAPT services:** The NHS offers Improving Access to Psychological Therapies (IAPT) services, which provide CBT-I as part of their offerings. You can self-refer to an IAPT service in your area, or your GP can refer you. Many IAPT services now offer online CBT-I programmes, which can be a convenient option.

Online CBT-I programmes:

- **Sleepio:** Sleepio is a popular, clinically validated online CBT-I programme available in the UK. It's designed to help you improve your sleep through a series of interactive sessions. You can access Sleepio through the NHS in some areas, or you may need to subscribe privately.
- **Sleepstation:** Another NHS-backed online CBT-I programme, Sleepstation provides personalised support to help you overcome insomnia. It's accessible with a referral from your GP, or you can sign up directly if you're looking for immediate help.

Private therapy:

Many therapists across the UK offer CBT-I, and you can find them through directories like the British Association for Behavioural and Cognitive Psychotherapies (BABCP) or through platforms like Psychology Today.

Progressive relaxation

Progressive muscle relaxation is an exercise that reduces stress and anxiety in your body by having you slowly tense and then relax each muscle. This exercise can provide an immediate feeling of relaxation, but it's best to practise frequently.

As you learn to do it, it can become a valuable tool to use when waking during the night. With experience, you will become more aware of when you're experiencing tension, and you will have the skills to help you relax. During this exercise, each muscle should be tensed but not to the point of strain. If you have any injuries or pain, you can skip the affected areas. Pay special attention to the feeling of releasing tension in each muscle and the resulting feeling of relaxation.

There are many versions of this online so feel free to try different ones so that you feel comfortable with the one you choose. I have also recorded a 20-minute script on my website.

How to do progressive relaxation

If you are practising during the day, sit back or lie down in a comfortable position. Shut your eyes if you are comfortable doing so.

If you are practising in your bed at night, firstly spend some time exploring your senses.

What does the air in the room feel like? Is it too warm, is it too cold or is it just OK?

What can you hear? Just observe the sounds, don't engage with them, they are what they are.

How does your bed feel? Are you cosy? Are the sheets comfortable and the pillow soft? Make any reasonable adjustments that you need to make to be comfortable.

How light is the room? For now just observe, it is what it is, but pay attention during the day to make sure that your room is sufficiently dark.

Begin by taking a deep breath and noticing the feeling of filling your lungs. Hold your breath for a few seconds.

5-second pause
Release the breath slowly and let the tension leave your body.

Take another deep breath and hold it.

5-second pause
Again, slowly release the air.

Even slower now, take another breath. Fill your lungs and hold the air.

5-second pause
Slowly release the breath and imagine the feeling of tension leaving your body.

Now, move your attention to your feet. Begin to tense your feet by curling your toes and the arch of your feet. Hold on to the tension and notice what it feels like.

5-second pause

Release the tension in your feet. Notice the new feeling of relaxation.

Next, begin to focus on your lower legs. Tense the muscles in your calves. Hold them tightly and pay attention to the feeling of tension.

5-second pause

Release the tension from your lower legs. Again, notice the feeling of relaxation. Remember to continue taking deep breaths.

Next, tense the muscles of your upper legs and pelvis. You can do this by tightly squeezing your thighs together. Make sure you feel tenseness without going to the point of strain.

5-second pause

And release. Feel the tension leave your muscles.

Begin to tense your stomach and chest. You can do this by sucking your stomach in; squeeze harder and hold the tension.

5-second pause

Release the tension. Allow your body to go limp. Let yourself notice the feeling of relaxation.

Continue taking deep breaths. Breathing slowly, fill your lungs and hold it.

5-second pause

Release the air slowly.

Next, tense the muscles in your back by bringing your shoulders together behind you. Hold them tightly. Tense them as hard as you can without straining and keep holding.

5-second pause

Release the tension from your back. Feel the tension slowly leaving your body, and then your feeling of relaxation. Notice how different your body feels when you allow it to relax.

Tense your arms all the way from your hands to your shoulders. Make a fist and squeeze all the way up your arm. Hold it.

5-second pause

Release the tension from your arms and shoulders. Notice the feeling of relaxation in your fingers, hands, arms and shoulders. Notice how your arms feel limp and at ease.

Move up to your neck and your head. Tense your face and your neck by squeezing the muscles around your eyes and mouth together.

5-second pause

Release the tension. Again, notice the new feeling of relaxation.

Finally, tense your whole body. Tense your feet, legs, tummy, chest, arms, head and neck. Tense harder without straining. Hold the tension.

5-second pause

Now release. Allow your whole body to go limp. Pay attention to the feeling of relaxation, and how different it is from the feeling of tension. Now that your body is relaxed, hopefully, it will help you to sleep. However, if you are still wide awake, get out of bed and go and read quietly or do something else until you feel tired.

Books and self-help resources:

Insomnia

There are also self-help books and resources that guide you through CBT-I techniques. *Overcoming Insomnia and Sleep Problems* by Professor Colin Espie is widely recommended.

Hello Sleep by Dr Jade Wu is an excellent resource. This book delves into the science behind sleep and insomnia, offering practical, evidence-based techniques for overcoming sleep difficulties without relying on medication.

Another excellent and highly recommended resource, which uses mindfulness and acceptance-based techniques, is *The Sleep Book* by Dr Guy Meadows. Dr Meadows, co-founder of The Sleep School, has drawn on his extensive expertise in sleep science and cognitive behavioural therapy to create a step-by-step approach for beating insomnia.

While not a substitute for personalised therapy, these resources can be a helpful starting point.

Narcolepsy

Julie Flygare's *Wide Awake and Dreaming* offers a deeply personal and illuminating journey into the world of narcolepsy, a misunderstood and often misdiagnosed sleep disorder. This memoir is both inspiring and educational, blending Flygare's story of living with narcolepsy with a broader understanding of the condition.

Sleep terrors and nightmares

In *Night Terrors*, Alice Vernon offers a fascinating exploration into the mysterious and unsettling world of sleep disorders. Drawing from her own experiences and extensive research, Vernon delves into the eerie phenomena of night terrors, sleep paralysis and other sleep disturbances, providing both a personal and scientific perspective.

Burnout

Claire Plumbly's *Burnout: How to Manage Your Nervous System Before It Manages You* offers a compassionate and insightful exploration of a topic that resonates with so many in our fast-paced, high-pressure world. With a blend of scientific understanding and practical strategies, Dr Plumbly provides readers with the tools to recognise the warning signs of burnout and take proactive steps to restore balance.

Yoga nidra and non-sleep deep rest (NSDR)

Unlike traditional mindfulness meditation, which often involves sitting alone in silence with closed eyes – an approach that may not be suitable for those facing significant stress or trauma – yoga nidra offers several advantages. First, you are lying down, making it generally more relaxing.

Second, you are not in a fully awake state; you are closer to the state of hypnagogia, naturally promoting physical relaxation. Third, the presence of the guided audio track means you are not alone with your thoughts, especially during challenging times.

Keep a selection of links in a specific place on your device so you know where to access them. They can be done lying down or sitting up. Set a timer if you fall asleep during practice.

It's important to explore these links during the day to see what appeals to you. There is no point using something for the first time at night and then finding you can't get on with it – you will tell me it doesn't work! It's not that it doesn't work. It's just that your brain isn't used to it, and when you cannot sleep, your ability to be rational about your choices is vastly reduced.

Note: Treat your device as a tool. Please turn off all notifications, use night-time filters and only use the device to access these tools.

NSDR (non-sleep deep rest) and yoga nidra are relaxation techniques but have similar origins, practices and purposes. Here's a breakdown:

NSDR (non-sleep deep rest):
Definition: The term NSDR is becoming more well-known due to the podcasts by Professor Andrew Huberman. Generally, NSDR refers to any practice or method enabling an individual to achieve deep rest without sleeping. It encompasses a variety of techniques designed to promote profound relaxation while keeping the practitioner conscious.

Purpose: NSDR techniques are primarily aimed at allowing individuals to rest and rejuvenate, especially if they're feeling fatigued but don't want to or can't fall asleep.

Techniques: NSDR can encompass various relaxation methods, such as guided imagery, deep breathing exercises or even specific meditation practices that don't specifically induce sleep.

Yoga nidra:
Definition: Yoga nidra, often called 'yogic sleep', is an ancient Indian relaxation practice that brings about conscious deep rest. It's a structured method that usually involves guided meditation.

Purpose: While deep relaxation is a primary goal, yoga nidra also seeks to bridge the conscious and subconscious mind. It can be used for various purposes, including stress reduction, emotional healing, and manifesting personal intentions or goals.

Techniques: A typical yoga nidra session involves lying in a comfortable position and being guided through instructions. These often start with body awareness and progressive relaxation, then move to guided visualisations and other deepening practices. The session usually ends by revisiting the practitioner's initial intention or sankalpa.

State of consciousness: Although it's termed 'yogic sleep', the goal of yoga nidra is not always to fall asleep. Instead, the practitioner remains in a liminal state between wakefulness and sleep, similar to the hypnagogic state. This allows for deep rest while maintaining a thread of conscious awareness.

In comparison:

Origins: NSDR is a broader, more general term that can include various relaxation techniques, while yoga nidra is a specific practice rooted in the yogic tradition.

Structure: Yoga nidra has a more structured format, typically following a specific sequence of stages to achieve its unique state of conscious relaxation. NSDR might be more varied in its techniques and approaches.

Goal: While both aim for deep relaxation, yoga nidra often incorporates spiritual or personal growth components, like setting intentions or addressing deep-seated beliefs.

Recommendations

These are links I recommend and there are more on my website. But different people like different approaches. Both Spotify and Apple Music have lots of versions. While this is a range of links to try, there are many more out there. Choose what works for you, then try it during one of your nap periods. You can do any of them as often as you like.

A guided 15-minute yoga nidra audio track from Ally Boothroyd: https://www.youtube.com/watch?v=cj_dqTBq4Ls&ab_channel=Ally Boothroyd per cent7CSarovaraYoga

This version is from Professor Andrew Huberman and Rory Cordial: https://www.youtube.com/watch?v=pL02HRFk2vo&ab_channel=Ma defor

Guided 20-minute yoga nidra audio track from Jennifer Piercy: https://insighttimer.com/jenniferpiercy/guided-meditations/yoga-ni dra-for-sleep

Guided 20-minute yoga nidra audio track from iRest founder Dr Richard Miller: https://www.youtube.com/watch?v=Psl9FKh6qPg

Guided 35-minute track from Yoga Nidra Network especially for falling asleep: https://www.yoganidranetwork.org/nidras/yoga-nidra-for-a-good -night-sleep/

A searchable database of Yoga Nidra Network sessions, giving you access to literally hundreds of different guided audios: https://www .yoganidranetwork.org/nidras

Support

Every Mind Matters. An NHS resource about sleep: www.nhs.uk/every -mind-matters/mental-health-issues/sleep

Professional associations

American Academy of Sleep Medicine (AASM). A professional society dedicated to sleep medicine, offering resources for professionals and the public: www.aasm.org

British Sleep Society. Promotes sleep research and education in the UK: www.sleepsociety.org.uk

Australian Sleep Health Foundation. Promotes sleep health awareness and education across Australia: www.sleephealthfoundation.org.au

Charities

The Sleep Charity. The Sleep Charity, incorporating The Sleep Council, provides advice and support to empower the nation to sleep better: www.thesleepcharity.org.uk

Mind. Bringing together an unstoppable network of individuals and communities – people who care about mental health to make a difference: www.mind.org.uk

Hope 2 Sleep. Support and advice on all things sleep apnea: www.hope2sleep.co.uk

Sleep Apnoea provide advice and support on sleep apnea: www.sleep-apnoea-trust.org

Narcolepsy UK. Supporting people with narcolepsy, cataplexy and idiopathic hypersomnia, their families, carers and others interested in improving their quality of life: www.narcolepsy.org.uk

Hypersomnolence UK. Extensive information on idiopathic hypersomnolence: www.hypersomnolence.org.uk

Young Minds. The UK's leading charity fighting for a world where no young person feels alone with their mental health: www.youngminds.org.uk

Non-profit organisations

Circadian Sleep Disorders Network. An independent nonprofit organisation dedicated to improving the lives of people with chronic circadian rhythm disorders: www.circadiansleepdisorders.org

RLS-UK. Supporting people with restless legs syndrome and periodic limb movement disorder: www.rls-uk.org

Other support

Working with nightmares
Dr Justin Havens offers a comprehensive set of self-help resources for resolving all types of nightmares at www.stopnightmares.org including a five-minute YouTube animation (https://youtu.be/q6oeg15KVAk) on how to work with nightmares.

Learn how to lucid dream

Charlie Morley has created a range of online video courses including lucid dreaming practices, but also the innovative new techniques of mindfulness of dream and sleep, the holistic approach to lucidity training, which Charlie co-created with meditation expert Rob Nairn: www .charliemorley.com

Endnotes

Introduction

1. Klein, S. (2009). *The Secret Pulse of Time: Making Sense of Life's Scarcest Commodity*. London: Hachette.

2. Walters, M. (2023). 'This 21-year-old recent grad just went viral for crying about her 9-to-5 job', *Glamour*, 1 November. Available at: https://www.glamour.com/story/this-21-year-old-recent-grad-just -went-viral-for-crying-about-her-9-to-5-job

3. The sleepy girl mocktail is a homemade beverage that gained popularity on TikTok as a sleep aid. First introduced by Calee Shea in January 2023, it was Gracie Norton, another content creator, who propelled it into the spotlight, making it viral that year. This alcohol-free drink typically combines calming, natural ingredients like tart cherry juice, known for its melatonin content, and magnesium, which helps relax muscles. It's possible that some of its positive effect is placebo – not a criticism because the mind–body connection is powerful. A belief in the mocktail's efficacy could trigger a relaxation response, aiding sleep. Added to that, the ritual of preparing and consuming the mocktail might promote a state of calm and readiness for sleep, demonstrating the impact of psychological factors.

4. Walker, M. (2017). *Why We Sleep: The New Science of Sleep and Dreams*. London: Penguin Books.

5. Huberman, A. (2023). 'Dr Matthew Walker: The science & practice of perfecting your sleep', *Huberman Lab*. Available at: https://www .hubermanlab.com/episode/dr-matthew-walker-the-science-and -practice-of-perfecting-your-sleep

6. Association for Psychological Science (2021). 'Spark Creativity with Thomas Edison's Napping Technique', *Association for Psychological*

Science. Available at: https://www.psychologicalscience.org/news /spark-creativity-with-thomas-edisons-napping-technique.html
Baldwin, N. (1995). *Edison: Inventing the Century*. Chicago: University of Chicago Press.

Chapter 1

1. Konnikova, M. (2015). 'The work we do while we sleep', *The New Yorker*, 8 July. Available at: https://www.newyorker.com/science/maria -konnikova/the-work-we-do-while-we-sleep
2. This is a rare occurrence, and if you are one, I wouldn't expect you to have picked up this book. Only about 1–3 per cent of the population are true genetic short sleepers, meaning their bodies naturally require significantly less sleep – usually around 4–6 hours per night – without any negative impact on their health or cognitive function. These individuals have a genetic mutation in the DEC2 gene that allows them to thrive on less sleep, a trait most of us don't share.
3. Borbély A. A. (1982). 'A two process model of sleep regulation', *Human Neurobiology*, 1(3), 195–204. PMID: 7185792.
4. Borbély, A. A. and Achermann, P. (1998). 'Homeostasis of human sleep', *Handbook of Behavioural State Control: Cellular and Molecular Mechanisms*, Boca Raton, FL: CRC Press.
5. Freeman, J. R., Saint-Maurice, P. F., Watts, E. L., Moore, S. C., Shams-White, M. M., Wolff-Hughes, D. L., Russ, D. E., Almeida, J. S., Caporaso, N. E., Hong, H. G., Loftfield, E. and Matthews, C. E. (2024). 'Actigraphy-derived measures of sleep and risk of prostate cancer in the UK Biobank', *Journal of the National Cancer Institute*, 116(3), 434–444. Available at: https://pubmed.ncbi.nlm.nih.gov/38013591/
6. Carskadon, M. A. and Dement, W. C. (2011). 'Monitoring and staging human sleep', in M. H. Kryger, T. Roth and W. C. Dement (eds), *Principles and Practice of Sleep Medicine*, 5th edn, St. Louis, MO: Elsevier Saunders.
7. Edinger, J. D., Bonnet, M. H., Bootzin, R. R., Doghramji, K., Dorsey, C. M., Espie, C. A., Jamieson, A. O., McCall, W. V., Morin, C. M. and Stepanski, E. J. (2000). 'Derivation of research diagnostic criteria for insomnia: Report of an American Academy of Sleep Medicine work group', *Sleep*, 23(8), 1073–1077. Available at: https://pubmed.ncbi.nlm .nih.gov/15683149/

8. Boulos, M. I., Jairam, T., Kendzerska, T., Im, J., Mekhael, A. and Murray, B. J. (2019). 'Normal polysomnography parameters in healthy adults: a systematic review and meta-analysis', *The Lancet Respiratory Medicine*, 7(6), 533–543. Available at: https://doi.org/10.1016/s2213 -2600(19)30057-8

9. Waterhouse, J., Fukuda, Y. and Morita, T. (2012). 'Daily rhythms of the sleep–wake cycle', *Journal of Physiological Anthropology*, 31(1), 5. Available at: https://pubmed.ncbi.nlm.nih.gov/22738268/

10. Blumberg, M. S., Lesku, J. A., Libourel, P. A., Schmidt, M. H. and Rattenborg, N. C. (2020). 'What is REM sleep?', *Current Biology*, 30(1), R38–R49. Available at: https://pubmed.ncbi.nlm.nih.gov /31910377/

11. Walker, M. P. and Helm, E. v. d. (2009). 'Overnight therapy? the role of sleep in emotional brain processing', *Psychological Bulletin*, 135(5), 731–748. Available at: https://doi.org/10.1037/a0016570

12. Sloan, M., Bourgeois, J. A., Leschziner, G., Pollak, T. A., Pitkanen, M., Harwood, R., Bosley, M., Bortoluzzi, A., Andreoli, L., Diment, W., Brimicombe, J., Ubhi, M., Barrere, C., Naughton, F., Gordon, C. and D'Cruz, D. (2024). 'Neuropsychiatric prodromes and symptom timings in relation to disease onset and/or flares in SLE: results from the mixed methods international INSPIRE study', *The Lancet*, 73, 102634. Available at: https://www.thelancet.com/action/showPdf?pii =S2589-5370 per cent2824 per cent2900213-X

13. Stickgold, R., Whidbee, D., Schirmer, B., Patel, V. and Hobson, J. A. (2000). 'Visual discrimination task improvement: A multi-step process occurring during sleep', *Journal of Cognitive Neuroscience*, 12(2), 246–254. Available at: https://pubmed.ncbi.nlm.nih.gov /10771409/

14. Walker, M. P. and van der Helm, E. (2009). 'Overnight therapy? The role of sleep in emotional brain processing', *Psychological Bulletin*, 135(5), 731–748. Available at: https://www.ncbi.nlm.nih.gov/pmc /articles/PMC2890316/

15. Therapy options for nightmares include imagery rehearsal therapy (IRT), eye movement desensitisation and reprocessing (EMDR), lucid dreaming therapy, hypnosis, and self-exposure therapy, which is often incorporated into cognitive behavioural therapy (CBT). These approaches aim to reduce the frequency and intensity of nightmares

by addressing underlying emotional triggers, helping individuals process trauma, and teaching strategies to reshape and control distressing dreams.

16. To learn more about Dr Justin Havens and how to work with the Dream Completion Technique® in full (the example I have illustrated is a somewhat truncated version), visit www.stopnightmares.org

Chapter 2

1. Winter, C. (2024) 'Insomnia and fear: So scared to sleep', Sleep Unplugged, episode 85 [Audio podcast]. Available at: https://www.youtube.com/watch?v=zZ4rK_IsZA8

2. Ohayon, M. M. et al. (1996). 'Hypnagogic and hypnopompic hallucinations: Pathological phenomena?', *British Journal of Psychiatry*, 169(4), 459–467. Available at: https://pubmed.ncbi.nlm.nih.gov/8894197/

3. Yount, G., Stumbrys, T., Koos, K., Hamilton, D. and Wahbeh, H. (2024). 'Decreased posttraumatic stress disorder symptoms following a lucid dream healing workshop', *Traumatology*, 30(4), 550–558. Available at: https://doi.org/10.1037/trm0000456. In fact, by the end of the sixth day of the study, over 85 per cent of the participants were no longer classified as having post traumatic stress disorder (using the self-report PTSD Checklist for *DSM*-5).

4. Dresler, M., Wehrle, R., Spoormaker, V. I., Koch, S. P., Holsboer, F. et al. (2011). 'Neural correlates of dream lucidity obtained from contrasting lucid versus non-lucid REM sleep: a combined EEG/fMRI case study', *Current Biology*, 21(7), 595–600. Available at: https://www.ncbi.nlm.nih.gov/pmc/articles/PMC3369221/

5. Exploding head syndrome is considered harmless and not indicative of any serious neurological or health issue. See Sachs, C. and Svanborg, E. (1991). 'The exploding head syndrome: polysomnographic recordings and therapeutic suggestions', *Sleep*, 14(3), 263–266. Available at: https://doi.org/10.1093/sleep/14.3.263

6. Vernon, A. (2022). *Night Terrors: Troubled Sleep and the Stories We Tell About It*. London: Icon Books.

7. Hilditch, C. J. and McHill, A. W. (2019). 'Sleep Inertia: Current Insights', *Nature and Science of Sleep*, 11, 155–165. Available at: https://doi.org/10.2147/nss.s188911

8. Stampi, C. (ed.). (1992). *Why We Nap: Evolution, Chronobiology, and Functions of Polyphasic and Ultrashort Sleep*. Boston, MA: Birkhäuser. Available at: https://link.springer.com/book/10.1007/978-1-4757 -2210-9

9. Yetish, G., Kaplan, H., Gurven, M., Wood, B. M., Pontzer, H., Manger, P. R., Wilson, C. L., McGregor, R. L. and Siegel, J. M. (2015). 'Natural sleep and its seasonal variations in three pre-industrial societies', *Current Biology*, 25(21), 2862–2868. Available at: https://doi .org/10.1016/j.cub.2015.09.046

10. Spurgeon, D. (2002). 'People who sleep for seven hours a night live longest', *BMJ*, 324(7335), 446. Available at: https://doi: 10.1136/bmj .324.7335.446.

11. Harvey, A. G. and Buysse, D. J. (2018). *Treating Sleep Problems, A Transdiagnostic Approach*. New York: Guildford Press.

12. National Institutes of Health (2018). 'Sleep deprivation increases Alzheimer's protein', *NIH Research Matters*, 24 April. Available at: https://www.nih.gov/news-events/nih-research-matters/sleep -deprivation-increases-alzheimers-protein

13. Ibid.

14. Piller, C. (2022). 'Potential fabrication in research images threatens key theory of Alzheimer's disease', *Science*, 21 July. Available at: https://www.science.org/content/article/potential-fabrication -research-images-threatens-key-theory-alzheimers-disease

15. Straits Research (2021). 'Sleep market size, share & trends analysis report by product type (smart bedding, lab services, apnea devices, medication, wearable devices, others), by indication (insomnia, sleep apnea, narcolepsy, restless leg syndrome, REM sleep behaviour disorder, others) and by region (North America, Europe, APAC, Middle East and Africa, LATAM): forecasts, 2021–2031'. Available at: https://straitsresearch.com/report/sleep-market

16. Baron, K. G., Abbott, S., Jao, N., Manalo, N. and Mullen, R. (2017). 'Orthosomnia: are some patients taking the quantified self too far?', *Journal of Clinical Sleep Medicine*, 13(2), 351–354. Available at: https://doi.org/10.5664/jcsm.6472

17. Gigli, G. L. and Valente, M. (2013). 'Should the definition of "sleep hygiene" be antedated by a century? A historical note based on an old book by Paolo Mantegazza', *Neurological Sciences*, 34(5), 755–760.

18. Mercier, C. (1890). *Sanity and Insanity*. London: Walter Scott Publishing Co.
19. Posner, D. (2011). 'Sleep hygiene', in Perlis, M., Aloia, M. and Kuhn, B. (eds), *Behavioural Treatments for Sleep Disorders*. London: Elsevier, pp. 31–43. Available at: https://doi.org/10.1016/b978-0-12-381522-4.00003-1
20. De Pasquale, C., El Kazzi, M., Sutherland, K., Shriane, A. E., Vincent, G. E., Cistulli, P. A. and Bin, Y. S. (2024). 'Sleep hygiene – what do we mean? a bibliographic review', *Sleep Medicine Reviews*, 75, 101930. Available at: https://doi.org/10.1016/j.smrv.2024.101930
21. Every Mind Matters (n.d.) 'Simple tips for better sleep' [video]. YouTube. Available at: https://www.youtube.com/watch?v=OvQTjAlIvI8
22. Ekirch, A. R. (2006). *At Day's Close: A History of Night-time*. London: Weidenfeld & Nicolson.
    Ekirch, A. R. (2018). 'What sleep research can learn from history', *Sleep Health: Journal of the National Sleep Foundation*, 4(6), 515–518. Available at: https://pubmed.ncbi.nlm.nih.gov/30442319/
    Ekirch, A. R. (2024). 'Additional Historical References to "Segmented Sleep"'. Available at: https://sites.google.com/vt.edu/roger-ekirch/sleep-research/segmented-sleep
23. It's important to note that while many people manage the shifts during Ramadan without major disruptions, others may experience short-term sleep deprivation, leading to increased daytime sleepiness or reduced alertness. However, these effects tend to resolve once normal routines are resumed after Ramadan.
24. Yetish, G., Kaplan, H., Gurven, M., Wood, B., Pontzer, H., Manger, P. R., Wilson, C., McGregor, R. and Siegel, J. M. (2015). 'Natural sleep and its seasonal variations in three pre-industrial societies', *Current Biology*, 25(21), 2862–2868. Available at: https://pubmed.ncbi.nlm.nih.gov/26480842/
25. Rosenblum, Y., Weber, F. D., Rak, M. et al. (2023). 'Sustained polyphasic sleep restriction abolishes human growth hormone release', *Sleep*, 47(2). Available at: https://doi.org/10.1093/sleep/zsad321
26. Ibid.
27. Cannon, J. (2023). 'By sleeping when everyone else is awake, I cured my insomnia', *Guardian*, 31 December. Available at: https://www.the

guardian.com/lifeandstyle/2023/dec/31/by-sleeping-when-everyone
-else-is-awake-i-cured-my-insomnia-joanna-cannon

28. Adapted from Harvey, A. G. and Buysse, D. J. (2018). *Treating Sleep Problems, A Transdiagnostic Approach*. New York: Guilford Press.

29. This routine draws on the research and methods presented by Harvey and Buysse (2018, see Note 28 above) in their transdiagnostic approach to treating sleep disorders. By incorporating these strategies into your morning routine, you can steadily enhance your sleep quality and overall wellbeing.

30. Roenneberg, T., Allebrandt, K. V., Merrow, M. and Vetter, C. (2012), 'Social jetlag and obesity', *Current Biology*, 22(10), 939–943. Available at: https://pubmed.ncbi.nlm.nih.gov/22578422//

31. Arab, A., Karimi, E., Garaulet, M. and Scheer, F. A. (2023). 'Social jetlag and dietary intake: a systematic review', *Sleep Medicine Reviews*, 71, 101820. Available at: https://pubmed.ncbi.nlm.nih.gov/37544031/

Chapter 3

1. The biopsychosocial (BPS) model was developed by psychiatrist George Engel in 1977 as a response to the limitations of the traditional biomedical model. Engel introduced the BPS model to provide a more holistic understanding of health and illness. The traditional biomedical model focused primarily on biological factors, treating the body as a machine that needed repairs when something went wrong. Engel argued that this approach was too narrow and failed to account for the psychological and social dimensions of health.
Engel's BPS model posits that health and illness result from the complex interplay of biological, psychological and social factors. Biological factors include genetics, physiology and biochemistry. Psychological factors encompass emotions, thoughts, behaviours and mental health. Social factors involve relationships, socioeconomic status, culture and environmental influences.
By integrating these three dimensions, the BPS model offers a more comprehensive approach to understanding and treating health issues. It recognises that a person's mental and social conditions significantly impact their physical health and vice versa. This model has since been

widely adopted in various fields, including medicine, psychology and healthcare, promoting a more holistic and patient-centred approach to health and wellbeing.

2. Walker, M. (2017). *Why We Sleep: Unlocking the Power of Sleep and Dreams.* New York: Scribner.

3. Sansone, R. A. and Sansone, L. A. (2012). 'Rumination: Relationships with physical health', *Innovations in Clinical Neuroscience*, 9(2), 29–34. Available at: https://www.ncbi.nlm.nih.gov/pmc/articles /PMC3312901

4. Cryan, J. F., O'Riordan, K. J., Cowan, C. S. M., Sandhu, K. V., Bastiaanssen, T. F. S., Boehme, M., Codagnone, M. G., Stilling, R. M., Borre, Y. E., Maguire, M., Moloney, G., Grosse, J. I., Mahony, S. M., Clarke, G. and Dinan, T. G. (2019). 'The microbiota–gut–brain axis', *Physiological Reviews*, 99(4), 1877–2013. Available at: https://doi: 10.1152/physrev.00018.2018.

5. Miles-Novelo, A. and Anderson, C. A. (2023). 'Climate crisis and aggression', *Psychology Today*. Available at: https://www.psychology today.com/us/blog/science-and-sensibility/202308/climate-crisis -and-aggression.

6. American Psychological Association (2023). 'Understanding anger'. Available at: https://www.apa.org/topics/anger.

7. Henry Ford Health (2023). 'Why does everyone seem so angry all of a sudden?' Henry Ford Health. Available at: https://www.henryford .com/blog/2023/03/why-does-everyone-seem-so-angry

8. Levine, P. A. (1997). *Waking the Tiger: Healing Trauma: The Innate Capacity to Transform Overwhelming Experiences.* Berkeley, CA: North Atlantic Books. This book introduces Levine's theories on how animals instinctively discharge trauma and reset their nervous systems – a foundational concept in his approach to trauma therapy, known as somatic experiencing. If you're looking for more recent sources or peer-reviewed articles, you may also want to explore Levine's later works or articles published by practitioners of somatic experiencing, as the concepts have been widely discussed and expanded upon in the field of trauma therapy.

9. Ibid.
Levine, P. A. (2010). *In an Unspoken Voice: How the Body Releases Trauma and Restores Goodness.* Berkeley, CA: North Atlantic Books.

10. Sanilevici, M., Reuveni, O., Lev-Ari, S., Golland, Y. and Levit-Binnun, N. (2021). 'Mindfulness-based stress reduction increases mental wellbeing and emotion regulation during the first wave of the COVID-19 pandemic: A synchronous online intervention study', *Frontiers in Psychology*, 12, 720965. Available at: https://doi: 10.3389/fpsyg.2021 .720965.

    Galante, J., Friedrich, C., Dawson, A. F., Modrego-Alarcón, M., Gebbing, P., Delgado-Suárez, I., Gupta, R., Dean, L., Dalgleish, T., White, I. R. and Jones, P. B. (2021). 'Mindfulness-based programmes for mental health promotion in adults in nonclinical settings: A systematic review and meta-analysis of randomised controlled trials', *PLOS Medicine*, 18(1), e1003481. Available at: https://doi: 10.1371 /journal.pmed.1003481.

11. Kabat-Zinn, J. (2017). 'Defining mindfulness'. Available at: https:// www.mindful.org/jon-kabat-zinn-defining-mindfulness/

12. While mindfulness has many benefits, it might not be the right fit for you for several reasons. If you have certain mental health conditions like severe depression, anxiety disorders or PTSD, mindfulness can sometimes exacerbate symptoms by bringing up distressing thoughts or memories. It might not align with your personal beliefs, cultural background or preferences, and you might find other practices more resonant. Practising mindfulness requires consistent effort and patience, which can be challenging if you struggle with concentration, have an active mind or are in an environment not conducive to quiet reflection. Misunderstanding mindfulness as merely a relaxation technique can lead to disillusionment if you don't achieve immediate results. Time commitment can be a barrier if you have a busy schedule or demanding responsibilities. If you are highly sensitive or have unresolved emotional issues, the increased awareness from mindfulness might cause emotional discomfort. Additionally, without proper guidance, you might struggle to practise effectively, leading to frustration. In acute crisis situations, more immediate interventions might be necessary, and alternative practices like physical exercise, creative activities or social interactions might be more beneficial for your wellbeing. Understanding that mindfulness is not a one-size-fits-all solution allows you to choose practices that best suit your individual needs and circumstances.

13. McKay, M., Wood, J. C. and Brantley, J. (2007). *The Dialectical Behavior Therapy Skills Workbook: Practical DBT Exercises for Learning Mindfulness, Interpersonal Effectiveness, Emotional Regulation and Distress Tolerance.* Oakland, CA: New Harbinger Publications.

14. Harris, A., Carmona, N. E., Moss, T. G. and Carney, C. E. (2020). 'Testing the contiguity of the sleep and fatigue relationship: A daily diary study', *Sleep*, 44(5). Available at: https://doi: 10.1093/sleep/zsaa252.

15. Levine (1997). *Waking the Tiger.*
    Levine (2010). *In an Unspoken Voice.*

16. Wegner, D. M. (1994). 'Ironic processes of mental control', *Psychological Review*, 101(1), 34–52. Available at: https://doi: 10.1037/0033-295x.101.1.34.

17. Colten, H. R. and Altevogt, B. M. (eds) (2006). *Sleep Disorders and Sleep Deprivation: An Unmet Public Health Problem.* Washington, DC: National Academies Press.

18. Yang, A. H., Palmer, A. A. and de Wit, H. (2010). 'Genetics of caffeine consumption and responses to caffeine', *Psychopharmacology*, 211(3), 245–257. Available at: http://doi: 10.1007/s00213-010-1900-1.

19. Ren, X. and Chen, J. (2020). 'Caffeine and Parkinson's disease: Multiple benefits and emerging mechanisms', *Frontiers in Neuroscience*, 14, 602697. Available at: https://:doi: 10.3389/fnins.2020.602697.

20. Drake, C., Roehrs, T., Shambroom, J. and Roth, T. (2013). 'Caffeine effects on sleep taken 0, 3, or 6 hours before going to bed', *Journal of Clinical Sleep Medicine*, 9(11), 1195–1200. Available at: https://jcsm.aasm.org/doi/10.5664/jcsm.3170

21. Thorn, C. F., Aklillu, E., McDonagh, E. M., Klein, T. E. and Altman, R. B. (2012). 'PharmGKB summary: Caffeine pathway', *Pharmacogenetics and Genomics*, 22(5), 389–395. doi: 10.1097/FPC.0b013e3283505d5e. Available at: https://www.ncbi.nlm.nih.gov/pmc/articles/PMC3381939/.

22. Research into the effects of caffeine on individuals with ADHD has shown mixed results. Several studies have examined whether caffeine can alleviate symptoms such as inattention and hyperactivity. A systematic review and meta-analysis found that while caffeine might help improve certain ADHD-related symptoms like inattention in some cases, it is generally less effective than traditional ADHD

medications like methylphenidate. Moreover, high doses of caffeine can sometimes worsen symptoms like impulsivity in both children and adults with ADHD.

Another study highlighted that caffeine's cognitive benefits, such as improved focus, might be limited, and the effects are often short-lived. Furthermore, caffeine's stimulant nature could potentially lead to anxiety or sleep issues, which may exacerbate ADHD symptoms rather than alleviate them.

However, some animal studies suggest caffeine may have potential as an adjuvant treatment for ADHD when used in lower doses, but these findings are still largely experimental and not widely supported for clinical use.

Given the inconsistent results, caffeine is not considered a reliable treatment for ADHD, and its effects can vary significantly between individuals. Anyone considering caffeine to manage ADHD should consult a healthcare professional.

23. Which? (2023). 'A little or a latte? – Which? finds huge differences in high-street coffee caffeine levels'. Available at: https://www.which.co.uk/policy-and-insight/article/a-little-or-a-latte-which-finds-huge-differences-in-high-street-coffee-caffeine-levels-athmJ0F9z1yS.

24. Planning Committee for a Workshop on Potential Health Hazards Associated with Consumption of Caffeine in Food and Dietary Supplements, Food and Nutrition Board, Board on Health Sciences Policy, Institute of Medicine (2014). 'Caffeine in food and dietary supplements: Examining safety: Workshop summary'. Washington, DC: National Academies Press (US).

25. Utter, J., Denny, S., Teevale, T. and Sheridan, J. (2018). 'Energy drink consumption among New Zealand adolescents: associations with mental health, health risk behaviours and body size', *Journal of Paediatrics and Child Health*, 54(3), 279–283. Available at: https://:doi:10.1111/jpc.13708.

26. Clarkson, J. (2023). *Clarkson's Farm* [TV series], Episode 5. Amazon Prime Video. Available at: http://www.amazon.com

27. Young, T., Skatrud, J. and Peppard, P. E. (2004). 'Risk factors for obstructive sleep apnea in adults', *JAMA*, 291(16), 2013–2016. Available at: https://doi.org/10.1001/jama.291.16.2013

28. Vitale, M., Costabile, G., Testa, R., D'Abbronzo, G., Nettore, I. C., Macchia, P. E. and Giacco, R. (2024). 'Ultra-processed foods and human health: a systematic review and meta-analysis of prospective cohort studies', *Advances in Nutrition*, 15(1), 100121. Available at: https://doi.org/10.1016/j.advnut.2023.09.009

29. Sadler, C., Grassby, T., Hart, K., Raats, M., Sokolović, M. and Timotijević, L. (2022). '"Even we are confused": a thematic analysis of professionals' perceptions of processed foods and challenges for communication', *Frontiers in Nutrition*, 9, 826162. Available at: https://doi.org/10.3389/fnut.2022.826162

30. Cappuccio, F. P., Taggart, F. M., Kandala, N. B., Currie, A., Peile, E., Stranges, S. and Miller, M. A. (2008). 'Meta-analysis of short sleep duration and obesity in children and adults', *Sleep*, 31(5), 619–626. Available at: https://doi.org/10.1093/sleep/31.5.619

31. Spiegel, K., Leproult, R., L'Hermite-Balériaux, M., Copinschi, G., Penev, P. D. and Cauter, E. V. (2004). 'Leptin levels are dependent on sleep duration: relationships with sympathovagal balance, carbohydrate regulation, cortisol, and thyrotropin', *Journal of Clinical Endocrinology and Metabolism*, 89(11), 5762–5771. Available at: https://doi.org/10.1210/jc.2004-1003

32. Roehrs, T. and Roth, T. (2001). 'Sleep sleepiness, sleep disorders and alcohol use and abuse', *Sleep Medicine Reviews*, 5(4), 287–297. Available at: https://pubmed.ncbi.nlm.nih.gov/12530993

Chapter 4

1. Kocevska, D., Blanken, T. F., Someren, E. J. V. and Rösler, L. (2020). 'Sleep quality during the Covid-19 pandemic: not one size fits all', *Sleep Medicine*, 76, 86–88. Available at: https://pubmed.ncbi.nlm.nih.gov/33126035/

2. Leone, M. J., Sigman, M. and Golombék, D. A. (2020). 'Effects of lockdown on human sleep and chronotype during the COVID-19 pandemic', *Current Biology*, 30(16), R930–R931. Available at: https://pubmed.ncbi.nlm.nih.gov/32810450/

3. Wood, Z. (2021). 'Lego doubles profits as demand soars beyond Covid-19 lockdown', *Guardian*, 28 September. Available at: https://www.theguardian.com/lifeandstyle/2021/sep/28/lego-profits-covid-19-lockdown-christmas-stock

4. Nielson-Stowell, A. (2022). 'Bubbling Over: Pandemic Sourdough', The Fermentation Association. Available at: https://fermentation association.org/bubbling-over-pandemic-sourdough/

5. Kalmbach, D. A., Schneider, L., Cheung, J., Bertrand, S. J., Kariharan, T., Pack, A. I. and Gehrman, P. (2016). 'Genetic basis of chronotype in humans: insights from three landmark GWAS', *Sleep*, 40(2). Available at: https://pubmed.ncbi.nlm.nih.gov/28364486/

6. The Daylight Site (n.d.). 'Body clocks, light, sleep and health'. [online] Available at: http://thedaylightsite.com/body-clocks-light-sleep-and -health/

7. The Nobel Prize in Physiology or Medicine (2017). 'Summary'. Available at: https://www.nobelprize.org/prizes/medicine/2017/summary/

8. Roenneberg, T., Wirz-Justice, A. and Merrow, M. (2007). 'Epidemiology of the human circadian clock', *Sleep Medicine Reviews*, 11(6), 429–38. Available at: https://pubmed.ncbi.nlm.nih.gov/17936039/

9. Meredith, N. (2019). 'Night owls can "retrain" their body clocks to improve mental well-being and performance', University of Surrey. Available at: https://www.surrey.ac.uk/news/night-owls-can-retrain -their-body-clocks-improve-mental-well-being-and-performance

10. Facer-Childs, E. R., Middleton, B., Skene, D. J. and Bagshaw, A. P. (2019). 'Resetting the late timing of "night owls" has a positive impact on mental health and performance', *Sleep Medicine*, 60, 236–247. Available at: https://pubmed.ncbi.nlm.nih.gov/31202686/

11. Typaldos, M. and Glaze, D. G. (2021). *Teenagers: Sleep Patterns and School Performance*. Available at: https://sleepeducation.org/wp-content /uploads/2021/04/teenssleeppatternsandschoolperformance.pdf

12. Klaufus, L., Verlinden, E., Wal, M. v. d., Cuijpers, P., Chinapaw, M. J. M. and Smit, F. (2022). 'Adolescent anxiety and depression: burden of disease study in 53,894 secondary school pupils in the Netherlands', *BMC Psychiatry*, 22(1), 225. Available at: https://doi.org/10.1186 /s12888-022-03868-5

13. Marx, R., Tanner-Smith, E. E., Davison, C. et al. (2017). 'Later school start times for supporting the education, health, and wellbeing of high school students', *Cochrane Database of Systematic Reviews*, 7. Available at: https://doi.org/10.1002/14651858.cd009467.pub2

14. Munich Chronotype Questionnaire (MCTQ): Roenneberg, T., Wirz-Justice, A. and Merrow, M. (2003). 'Life between clocks: daily

temporal patterns of human chronotypes', *Journal of Biological Rhythms*, 18(1), 80–90. Available at: https://doi.org/10.1177/0748730402239679.

15. Morningness-Eveningness Questionnaire (MEQ): Horne, J. A. and Ostberg, O. (1976). 'A self-assessment questionnaire to determine morningness-eveningness in human circadian rhythms', *International Journal of Chronobiology*, 4(2), 97–110.

16. Windred, D. P., Burns, A. C., Lane, J. M., Saxena, R., Rutter, M. K., Cain, S. W. and Phillips, A. J. K. (2023). 'Sleep regularity is a stronger predictor of mortality risk than sleep duration: a prospective cohort study', *Sleep*, 47(1). Available at: https://doi.org/10.1093/sleep/zsad253

17. Rosseinsky, K. (2023). 'Rishi Sunak reveals why he gets up at 5am and the part of the job he dreads the most', *Independent* [online]. Available at: https://www.independent.co.uk/life-style/rishi-sunak-sleep-wake-up-b2403404.html

18. Willett, W. (1907) *The Waste of Daylight*. London: Hazell, Watson and Viney.

19. Ghosh, P. (2016) 'The builder who changed how the world keeps time', *BBC Future*, 10 March. Available at: https://www.bbc.com/future/article/20160310-the-builder-who-changed-how-the-world-keeps-time

20. Zhang, H., Dahlén, T., Khan, A. A., Edgren, G. and Rzhetsky, A. (2020). 'Measurable health effects associated with the daylight saving time shift', *PLOS Computational Biology*, 16(6), e1007927. Available at: https://doi.org/10.1371/journal.pcbi.1007927

21. Prats-Uribe, A., Tobías, A. and Prieto-Alhambra, D. (2018). 'Excess risk of fatal road traffic accidents on the day of daylight saving time change', *Epidemiology*, 29, e44–e45. Available at: https://pubmed.ncbi.nlm.nih.gov/29864085/

22. Chaix, A., Manoogian, E. N. C., Melkani, G. C. and Panda, S. (2019). 'Time-restricted eating to prevent and manage chronic metabolic diseases', *Annual Review of Nutrition*, 39(1), 291–315. Available at: https://pubmed.ncbi.nlm.nih.gov/31180809/

23. Wilkinson, M. J., Manoogian, E. N. C., Zadourian, A., Lo, H., Fakhouri, S., Shoghi, A., Fleischer, J. G., Navlakha, S., Panda, S. and Taub, P. R. (2020). 'Ten-hour time-restricted eating reduces weight, blood pressure, and atherogenic lipids in patients with metabolic syndrome', *Cell Metabolism*, 31(1), 92–104.e5. Available at: https://pubmed.ncbi.nlm.nih.gov/31813824/

24. Time-restricted eating (TRE) isn't effective for everyone. It can be challenging for people with medical conditions like diabetes, individuals with eating disorders, pregnant or breastfeeding women, children, adolescents, older adults and high-performance athletes. A study by UC San Francisco found no significant difference in weight loss or metabolic health between those who practised TRE and those with regular meal timing. Additionally, TRE may lead to loss of lean muscle mass. Compliance with strict eating windows can also be difficult for people with irregular schedules. It's important to consult with a healthcare provider before starting TRE.

25. Danvers, A. F., Efinger, L. D., Mehl, M. R., Helm, P. J., Raison, C. L., Polsinelli, A. J., Moseley, S. A. and Sbarra, D. A. (2023). 'Loneliness and time alone in everyday life: a descriptive-exploratory study of subjective and objective social isolation', *Journal of Research in Personality*, 107, 104426. Available at: https://www.sciencedirect.com/ science/article/pii/S0092656623000880?via per cent3Dihub

26. Hirohama, K., Imura, T., Hori, T., Deguchi, N., Mitsutake, T. and Tanaka, R. (2024). 'The effects of nonpharmacological sleep hygiene on sleep quality in nonelderly individuals: A systematic review and network meta-analysis of randomised controlled trials', *PLOS One*, 19(6), p. e0301616. Available at: https://www.ncbi.nlm.nih.gov/pmc /articles/PMC11152306/

27. Mosley, M. (2018). 'Forget walking 10,000 steps a day', *BBC News*, 5 February. Available at: https://www.bbc.co.uk/news/health-42864061

28. McCurdy, C. and Murphy, L. (2024). 'We've only just begun: Action to improve young people's mental health, education and employment'. Resolution Foundation, February.

29. Building H. (n.d.). 'Survey Research' [online]. Available at: https:// www.buildingh.org/survey-research
Ritchie, H. (2023). 'A survey of modern life: Outdoor time', *Building H* [online]. Available at: https://medium.com/building-h/a-survey-of -modern-life-outdoor-time-3a99d9fa3acb

30. Auger, R. R., Burgess, H. J., Emens, J. S., Deriy, L. V., Thomas, S. M. and Sharkey, K. M. (2015). 'Clinical practice guideline for the treatment of intrinsic circadian rhythm sleep-wake disorders: advanced sleep-wake phase disorder (ASWPD), delayed sleep-wake phase disorder (DSWPD), non-24-hour sleep-wake rhythm disorder

(N24SWD), and irregular sleep-wake rhythm disorder (ISWRD). An update for 2015', *Journal of Clinical Sleep Medicine*, 11(10), 1199–1236. Available at: https://doi.org/10.5664/jcsm.5100

31. Blume, C., Garbazza., C, Spitschan, M. (2019). 'Effects of light on human circadian rhythms, sleep and mood', *Somnologie (Berl)*, 23(3), 147–156. Available at: doi: 10.1007/s11818-019-00215-x. PMID: 31534436; PMCID: PMC6751071.

32. Roenneberg, T., Wirz-Justice, A. and Merrow, M. (2003). 'Life between clocks: daily temporal patterns of human chronotypes', *Journal of Biological Rhythms*, 18(1), 80–90. Available at: https://pubmed.ncbi.nlm.nih.gov/12568247/

33. Shanahan, T. L. and Czeisler, C. A. (1991). 'Light exposure induces equivalent phase shifts of the endogenous circadian rhythms of circulating plasma melatonin and core body temperature in men', *Journal of Clinical Endocrinology & Metabolism*, 73(2), 227–235. Available at: https://pubmed.ncbi.nlm.nih.gov/1856258

34. Duffy, J. F. and Czeisler, C. A. (2009). 'Effect of light on human circadian physiology', *Sleep Medicine Clinics*, 4(2), 165–177. Available at: https://www.ncbi.nlm.nih.gov/pmc/articles/PMC2717723/

35. It's important to note that individual experiences may vary. Some people may have a strong preference for darkness without experiencing intense aversion or anxiety. Additionally, factors like sleep disorders, other health conditions and lifestyle habits can also influence sleep quality.

36. In clinical settings, melatonin is usually prescribed in small doses, typically between 0.5 and 3 milligrams. If you purchase an over-the-counter product that contains 5 milligrams or more, it may exceed the amount that is considered safe or effective for most people. Doctors generally recommend very low doses, taken one to two hours before bedtime, especially for those who struggle with falling asleep at a normal time. Taking melatonin at the wrong time or in too high a dose can actually worsen sleep problems by disrupting your circadian rhythm, rather than improving it.

37. Melatonin is often prescribed in specific cases, particularly for neurodiverse individuals, such as those with autism spectrum disorder (ASD) or attention deficit hyperactivity disorder (ADHD). It

is used to help manage sleep challenges, especially difficulties with falling asleep or disrupted sleep patterns. Its administration should be carefully tailored to the individual's needs and integrated into a comprehensive sleep management plan under the guidance of a healthcare professional.

38. Office for National Statistics (ONS). (2022). 'The night-time economy, UK: 2022'. Available at: https://www.ons.gov.uk/businessindustry andtrade/business/activitysizeandlocation/articles/thenighttime economyuk/2022

39. Scheer, F. A., Hilton, M. F., Mantzoros, C. S. and Shea, S.A. (2009). 'Adverse metabolic and cardiovascular consequences of circadian misalignment', *Proceedings of the National Academy of Sciences*, 106(11), 4453–4458. Available at: https://doi.org/10.1073/pnas.0808180106.

40. Department of Health and Social Care. (2022). 'Establishing food standards for NHS hospitals'. Available at: https://www.gov.uk /government/publications/establishing-food-standards-for-nhs -hospitals#:~:text=The%20report%20looks%20at%20standards,in %20the%20NHS%20in%20England

41. Shriane, A. E., Rigney, G., Ferguson, S. A., Bin, Y. S. and Vincent, G. E. (2023). 'Healthy sleep practices for shift workers: consensus sleep hygiene guidelines using a Delphi methodology', *Sleep*, 46(12). Available at: https://pubmed.ncbi.nlm.nih.gov/37429599/

42. Walker, M. (guest). (2023). 'The Drive with Peter Attia' [audio podcast]. Available at: https://peterattiamd.com/

43. Williams, J. (2018). *Stand Out of Our Light: Freedom and Resistance in the Attention Economy*. Cambridge: Cambridge University Press.

Chapter 5

1. Levine, P. A. (1997). *Waking the Tiger: Healing Trauma*. Berkeley, CA: North Atlantic Books.

2. While some critics contend that PVT oversimplifies the autonomic nervous system and lacks robust empirical support, its strength lies in illustrating how our physiological states shape psychological experiences and behaviours. As a psychotherapist, I find its practical applications invaluable, offering tools to help you understand and regulate both your physiological and psychological states. By

recognising where you are in the moment, this framework facilitates a more responsive and effective therapeutic process, empowering you to navigate challenges with greater awareness and adaptability.

3. For more about Deb Dana, visit her website and discover 'The science of feeling safe enough to fall in love with life'. Available at: https://www.rhythmofregulation.com

4. The vagal brake is a helpful metaphor that has resonated with many practitioners and clients for understanding the body's ability to regulate stress. However, as with many theories in neuroscience, it's a model that simplifies a very complex system. While it can be a powerful tool for teaching emotional regulation, it's important to recognise its limitations and remember that emotional health is influenced by many factors beyond the vagus nerve alone.

5. Hanson, R. (2013). 'Hardwiring Happiness', TEDxMarin, 17 September [online video]. Available at: https://www.youtube.com/watch?v=jpuDyGgIeh0

6. As a psychotherapist, I focus on integrating the body and mind to help clients navigate the unique challenges of hypersomnia. In situations like this, I work alongside other medical specialists to ensure comprehensive care. While my work emphasises nervous system regulation, and draws on other strategies like cognitive behavioural therapy (CBT) and making lifestyle adjustments (such as improving sleep hygiene and managing stress), when needed, medication plays an important role.

7. Martin-Gill C., Barger L. K., Moore C. G., Higgins J. S., Teasley E. M., Weiss P. M. et al. (2018). 'Effects of napping during shift work on sleepiness and performance in emergency medical services personnel and similar shift workers: a systematic review and meta-analysis', *Prehospital Emergency Care*, 22(sup1), 47–57. Available at: https://pubmed.ncbi.nlm.nih.gov/29324083/

8. Matsumoto K. and Harada, M. (1994). 'The effect of night-time naps on recovery from fatigue following night work', *Ergonomics*, 37(5), 899–907. Available at: https://pubmed.ncbi.nlm.nih.gov/8206058/

9. Patterson, P. D., Hilditch, C. J., Weaver, M. D., Roach, D. G., Okerman, T. S., Martin, S. E., . . . & Weiss, L. S. (2023). 'The effect of a night shift nap on post-night shift performance, sleepiness, mood, and first recovery sleep: a randomised crossover trial', *Scandinavian*

Journal of Work, Environment & Health, 50(1), 22–27. Available at: https://pmc.ncbi.nlm.nih.gov/articles/PMC10924715/

10. Mednick, S., Nakayama, K. and Stickgold, R. (2003). 'Sleep-dependent learning: a nap is as good as a night', *Nature Neuroscience*, 6, 697–698. Available at: https://www.nature.com/articles/nn1078

11. Maté, G. (2003). *When the Body Says No: The Cost of Hidden Stress*. Hoboken, NJ: Wiley.

12. Herman, J. L. (1992) *Trauma and Recovery: The Aftermath of Violence – From Domestic Abuse to Political Terror*. New York: Basic Books.

13. While irritable bowel syndrome (IBS) can often be influenced by psychological factors such as stress and anxiety, it's important to recognise that these symptoms might also signal other underlying medical conditions. Therefore, it's always advisable to consult a healthcare professional for a thorough evaluation. Getting it checked out ensures that any other potential causes are ruled out, and that you receive appropriate guidance and treatment.

14. While this idea is supported in some therapeutic modalities, like somatic therapy, trauma-focused therapy and body-focused psychotherapies, it is more controversial in mainstream psychology, where the extent and validity of somatic memory are still debated. Some may argue that the body does not literally 'remember' in the way the mind does, but that physical symptoms (like gut issues, muscle tension, or pain) can be linked to emotional or psychological stress, often unconsciously.

15. Sapolsky, R. M. (2004). *Why Zebras Don't Get Ulcers*. New York: St. Martin's Press.

16. Felitti, V. J., Anda, R. F., Nordenberg, D., Williamson, D. F., Spitz, A. M., Edwards, V., Koss, M. P., and Marks, J. S. (1998). 'Relationship of childhood abuse and household dysfunction to many of the leading causes of death in adults: The Adverse Childhood Experiences (ACE) Study', *American Journal of Preventive Medicine*, 14(4), 245–258. Available at: ttps://doi.org/10.1016/S0749-3797(98)00017-8

17. Wu, M., Chiao, C. and Lin, W. (2024). 'Adverse childhood experience and persistent insomnia during emerging adulthood: do positive childhood experiences matter?', *BMC Public Health*, 24(1). Available at: https://pubmed.ncbi.nlm.nih.gov/38267852/

18. Maslow, A. H. (1943). 'A theory of human motivation', *Psychological Review*, 50(4), 370–396.
    Maslow, A. H. (1954). *Motivation and Personality*. New York: Harper & Row. His theory emphasises security as a foundational need, but critics argue that his hierarchical structure doesn't fully capture the complexity of human experience, especially across different cultures. While his model offers valuable insight, current research suggests that human motivation is more nuanced and not easily organised into a rigid pyramid.

19. It originates from the work of Canadian psychologist Donald Hebb, who proposed the concept in his 1949 book, *The Organisation of Behaviour.*

20. Tubbs, A., Fernandez, F., Grandner, M., Perlis, M. L. and Klerman, E. B. (2022). 'The mind after midnight: nocturnal wakefulness, behavioural dysregulation, and psychopathology', *Frontiers in Network Physiology*, 1. Available at: https://www.ncbi.nlm.nih.gov /pmc/articles/PMC9083440/

21. Perlis, M. L., Grandner, M. A., Chakravorty, S., Bernert, R. A., Brown, G. K. and Thase, M. E. (2016). 'Suicide and sleep: Is it a bad thing to be awake when reason sleeps?', *Sleep Medicine Reviews*, 29, 101–107. doi:10.1016/j.smrv.2015.10.003

22. Jeffers, S. (1987). *Feel the Fear and Do It Anyway*. London: Arrow Books.

23. Clair Vickery used the term 'time poverty'. See Vickery, C. (1977). 'The Time-Poor: A New Look at Poverty', *Journal of Human Resources*, 12(1), 27–48. Available at: https://doi.org/10.2307/145597
    She used the term to describe the lack of time for leisure and personal activities experienced by individuals, particularly working women, due to the demands of their jobs and household responsibilities. Her work highlighted the challenges of balancing work and family life, and the resulting scarcity of time. See also Bailyn, L. (1980). 'Time poverty: the lack of time for leisure and personal activities', *Journal of Social Issues*, 36(4), 125–137.

24. Dalton-Smith, S. (2019). 'The real reason why we are tired and what to do about it', TED Talk, October. Available at: https://www.ted.com /talks/saundra_dalton_smith_the_real_reason_why_we_are_tired _and_what_to_do_about_it

25. Sakurada, K., Konta, T., Watanabe, M., Ishizawa, K., Ueno, Y. et al. (2020). 'Associations of frequency of laughter with risk of all-cause

mortality and cardiovascular disease incidence in a general population: findings from the Yamagata study', *Journal of Epidemiology*, 30(4), 188–193. Available at: https://pubmed.ncbi .nlm.nih.gov/30956258/

Chapter 6

1. Cohen, M. J. (n.d.). *Educating, Counselling and Healing With Nature Via 53 Natural Senses*. Available at: https://www.ecopsych.com /kechnarticle.html
2. Macomber, J. D. and Allen, J. G. (2020). 'We spend 90% of our time inside—why don't we care that indoor air is so polluted?', *Fast Company*, 20 May. Available at: https://www.fastcompany.com /90506856/we-spend-90-of-our-time-inside-why-dont-we-care-that -indoor-air-is-so-polluted
3. Nichols, W. J. (2014). *Blue Mind: The Surprising Science That Shows How Being Near, In, On, or Under Water Can Make You Happier, Healthier, More Connected, and Better at What You Do*. New York: Little, Brown and Company. Blue Mind promotes a mindful, relaxed state and provides a counter to 'Red Mind', which is characterised by stress, anxiety and a state of high alert due to the fast-paced, overstimulated nature of modern life. 'Grey Mind' is linked to feelings of depression, numbness and a lack of motivation, often resulting from prolonged exposure to stress and overstimulation.
4. Oishi, S., Talhelm, T. and Lee, M. (2015). 'Personality and geography: introverts prefer mountains', *Journal of Research in Personality*, 58, 55–68. Available at: https://www.sciencedirect.com/science/article /abs/pii/S0092656615300027
5. Schwichtenberg, A. J., Janis, A., Lindsay, H., Desai, A., Sahu, A., Kellerman, P. L. H., Abel, E. A. and Yatcilla, J. K. (2022). 'Sleep in children with autism spectrum disorder: A narrative review with recommendations for future research', *Current Developmental Disorders Reports*, 9(1), 1–11. Available at: https://doi.org/10.1007 /s40675-022-00234-5
Malow, B. A., Byars, K. C., Johnson, K., Weiss, S. K., Bernal, P., Goldman, S. E., Panzer, R., Coury, D. L. and Glaze, D. G. (2012). 'A practice pathway for the identification, evaluation, and management of insomnia in children and adolescents with autism spectrum

disorders', *Pediatrics*, 130(Supplement_2), S106-S124. Available at: https://doi.org/10.1542/peds.2012-0900i

6. Eye movement desensitisation and reprocessing (EMDR) is a psychotherapeutic approach that is primarily used to treat trauma and post-traumatic stress disorder (PTSD). Developed by Francine Shapiro in the late 1980s, EMDR involves the patient recalling distressing experiences while simultaneously undergoing bilateral sensory input, typically in the form of side-to-side eye movements.

7. Cirelli, C. and Tononi, G. (2015). 'Cortical development, electroencephalogram rhythms, and the sleep/wake cycle', *Biological Psychiatry*, 77(12), 1071–1078. Available at: https://pubmed.ncbi.nlm.nih.gov/25680672/

8. Basner, M., Müller, U. and Elmenhorst, E. M. (2014). 'Single and combined effects of air, road, and rail traffic noise on sleep and recuperation', *Sleep*, 37(11), 1421–1430. Available at: https://pubmed.ncbi.nlm.nih.gov/21203365/

9. Thoma, M. V., Marca, R. L., Brönnimann, R., Finkel, L., Ehlert, U. and Nater, U. M. (2013). 'The effect of music on the human stress response', *PLOS ONE*, 8(8), e70156. Available at: https://www.ncbi.nlm.nih.gov/pmc/articles/PMC3734071/

10. Carvell, S. (2020). 'White noise as sleep aid may do more harm than good, say scientists', *Guardian*, 18 October. Available at: https://www.theguardian.com/lifeandstyle/2020/oct/18/white-noise-as-sleep-aid-may-do-more-harm-than-good-say-scientists

11. Newcastle Hospitals NHS Foundation Trust (n.d.). 'Tinnitus and sleep disturbance'. Available at: https://www.newcastle-hospitals.nhs.uk/services/neurosciences/neurology/neurological-sleep-disorders/tinnitus-and-sleep-disturbance/

12. O'Connor, G. (dir.) (2016). *The Accountant* [film]. Warner Bros. Pictures.

13. Hayden, C. (2019). Facebook post, 10 April. Available at: https://www.facebook.com/chloeshayden/posts/autism-isnt-always-easyliving-in-a-world-that-wasnt-created-for-the-way-your-bra/1309043789236889/

14. Roberts, N. A., Burleson, M. H., Pituch, K. A., Flores, M., Woodward, C., Shahid, S., Todd, M. and Davis, M. C. (2022). 'Affective experience and regulation via sleep, touch, and "sleep-touch" among couples', *Journal of Affective Science*, 3(2), 353–369. Available at: https://www.ncbi.nlm.nih.gov/pmc/articles/PMC9382971/

15. Harvard Medical School (2020). 'Why stress causes people to overeat', *Harvard Health* [online]. Available at: https://www.health.harvard.edu /staying-healthy/why-stress-causes-people-to-overeat

16. van Egmond, L. T., Meth, E. M. S., Engström, J., Ilemosoglou, M., Keller, J. A., Vogel, H. and Benedict, C. (2023). 'Effects of acute sleep loss on leptin, ghrelin, and adiponectin in adults with healthy weight and obesity: A laboratory study', *Obesity (Silver Spring)*, 31(3), 635–641. Available at: https://pubmed.ncbi.nlm.nih.gov/36404495/

17. Leschziner, G. (2019). *The Nocturnal Brain: Nightmares, Neuroscience, and the Secret World of Sleep.* London: Simon & Schuster.

18. Dunbar, R. (2017). 'Breaking bread: the functions of social eating', *Adaptive Human Behaviour and Physiology*, 3(3), 198–211. Available at: https://pubmed.ncbi.nlm.nih.gov/32025474/

19. While these foods and drinks are often recommended for better sleep, their effectiveness may vary from person to person. They may help promote relaxation and contribute to a bedtime routine, which can be beneficial for sleep hygiene. However, they should not be relied upon as sole treatments for sleep disorders.

20. Nishitani, S., Miyamura, T., Tagawa, M., Sumi, M. et al. (2009). 'The calming effect of a maternal breast milk odour on the human newborn infant', *Neuroscience Research*, 63(1), 66–71. Available at: https://pubmed.ncbi.nlm.nih.gov/19010360/

21. Herz, R. S. and Engen, T. (1996). 'Odour memory: Review and analysis', *Psychonomic Bulletin & Review*, 3(3), 300–313. Available at: https://pubmed.ncbi.nlm.nih.gov/24213931/

22. Hofer, M. K., Collins, H. K., Whillans, A. V. and Chen, F. S. (2018). 'Olfactory cues from romantic partners and strangers influence women's responses to stress', *Journal of Personality and Social Psychology*, 114(1), 1–9. Available at: https://doi.org/10.1037 /pspa0000110

23. Tribunal de Grande Instance de Rennes (2019). Case involving noise pollution from wind turbines in Saint-Aubin-des-Châteaux, Loire-Atlantique, France, January.

24. Gallagher, M., Kearney, B. E. & Ferrè, E. R. (2021). 'Where is my hand in space? the internal model of gravity influences proprioception', *Biology Letters*, 17(6), 20210115. Available at: https://doi.org/10.1098 /rsbl.2021.0115

25. Ackerley, R., Olausson, H. and Badre, G. (2015). 'Positive effects of a weighted blanket on insomnia', *Journal of Sleep Medicine and Disorders*, 2, 1022. Available at: https://www.jscimedcentral.com /SleepMedicine/sleepmedicine-2-1022.pdf.

26. Mecking, O. (2021). *Niksen: Embracing the Dutch Art of Doing Nothing*. Boston, MA: Houghton Mifflin Harcourt.

27. Stallard, M. (2022). 'The breathing technique that can make you a better leader', *Yale Insights*. Available at: https://insights.som.yale.edu /insights/the-breathing-technique-that-can-make-you-better-leader

28. Jerath, R., Edry, J. W., Barnes, V. A. and Jerath, V. (2006). 'Physiology of long pranayamic breathing: Neural respiratory elements may provide a mechanism that explains how slow deep breathing shifts the autonomic nervous system', *Medical Hypotheses*, 67(3), 566–571. Available at: https://pubmed.ncbi.nlm.nih.gov/16624497/

29. van der Kolk, B. A. (2014). *The Body Keeps the Score: Brain, Mind, and Body in the Healing of Trauma*. New York: Viking.

30. Griffith, F. R. Jr., Pucher, G. W., Brownell, K. A., Klein, J. D. and Carmer, M. E. (1929). *Studies in Human Physiology III. Alveolar Air and Blood Gas Capacity*. Department of Physiology, University of Buffalo, Buffalo, NY.

31. Knutson, F. (2020). 'How to Enter the Theta State Anytime' [video]. YouTube. Available at: https://www.youtube.com/watch?v=J_2A-m -oeQU

Chapter 7

1. Ohayon, M. M., Carskadon, M. A., Guilleminault, C. and Vitiello, M. V. (2004). 'Meta-analysis of quantitative sleep parameters from childhood to old age in healthy individuals: developing normative sleep values across the human lifespan', *Sleep*, 27(7), 1255–1273. Available at: https://pubmed.ncbi.nlm.nih.gov/15164900/

2. Baker, F. C., Lampio, L., Saaresranta, T. and Polo-Kantola, P. (2018). 'Sleep and sleep disorders in the menopausal transition', *Sleep Medicine Clinics*, 13(3), 443–456. Available at: https://www.ncbi.nlm .nih.gov/pmc/articles/PMC6092036/

3. Kecklund, G. and Axelsson, J. (2016). 'Health consequences of shift work and insufficient sleep', *BMJ*, 355, i5210. Available at: https:// www.bmj.com/content/355/bmj.i5210

4. Roth, T. (2007). 'Insomnia: Definition, prevalence, etiology, and consequences', *Sleep Medicine Reviews*, 11(1), 1–9. Available at: https://www.ncbi.nlm.nih.gov/pmc/articles/PMC1978319

5. Hypersomnia Foundation (n.d.) 'What are hypersomnia sleep disorders?' Available at: https://www.hypersomniafoundation.org

6. Individuals with UARS may experience excessive daytime sleepiness, unrefreshing sleep, morning headaches and difficulty concentrating. UARS can be challenging to diagnose because standard sleep studies may not detect the subtle airway resistance increases. Specialised tests measuring oesophageal pressure changes are often needed. Similar to OSA, treatments may include continuous positive airway pressure (CPAP) therapy, oral appliances to keep the airway open or surgical interventions in some cases.

7. Young, T., Finn, L., Peppard, P. E., Szklo-Coxe, M., Austin, D., Nieto, F. J., Stubbs, R. and Hla, K. M. (2008). 'Sleep disordered breathing and mortality: eighteen-year follow-up of the Wisconsin sleep cohort', *Sleep*, 31(8), 1071–1078.

8. Steier, J., Martin, A.L., Harris, J., Jarrold, I., Pugh, D. and Williams, A. J. (2013). 'Predicted relative prevalence estimates for obstructive sleep apnea and the associated healthcare provision across the UK', *Thorax*, 69(4), 390–392. Available at: https://pubmed.ncbi.nlm.nih.gov/24062427/

9. Chung, F., Subramanyam, R., Liao, P., Sasaki, E., Shapiro, C. and Sun, Y. (2012). 'High STOP-Bang score indicates a high probability of obstructive sleep apnoea', *British Journal of Anaesthesia*, 108(5), 768–775. Available at: https://doi.org/10.1093/bja/aes022

10. Grigg-Damberger, M. (2016). 'The visual scoring of sleep in infants 0 to 2 months of age', *Journal of Clinical Sleep Medicine*, 12(3), 429–445. Available at: https://pubmed.ncbi.nlm.nih.gov/26951412/

11. Bathory, E. and Tomopoulos, S. (2017). 'Sleep regulation, physiology, and development', *Current Problems in Pediatric and Adolescent Health Care*, 47(2), 29–42. Available at: https://pubmed.ncbi.nlm.nih.gov/28117135/

12. Feldman, R. (2007) 'Parent–infant synchrony and the construction of shared timing: physiological precursors, developmental outcomes, and risk conditions', *Journal of Child Psychology and Psychiatry*, 48(3–4), 329–354. Available at: https://pubmed.ncbi.nlm.nih.gov/17355401/

13. World Health Organization. (2016). 'WHO recommendations on antenatal care for a positive pregnancy experience'. Available at: https://iris.who.int/bitstream/handle/10665/259947/WHO-RHR-18.02-eng.pdf

14. Bandura, A. (1977). *Social Learning Theory*. Englewood Cliffs, NJ: Prentice Hall.

15. Bowlby, J. (1988). *A Secure Base: Parent–Child Attachment and Healthy Human Development*. New York: Basic Books.

16. Porges, S. W. (2011). *The Polyvagal Theory: Neurophysiological Foundations of Emotions, Attachment, Communication, and Self-Regulation*. New York: W. W. Norton & Company.

17. Piaget, J. (1952). *The Origins of Intelligence in Children*. New York: International Universities Press.

18. Crowley, S. J., Acebo, C. and Carskadon, M. A. (2007). 'Sleep, circadian rhythms, and delayed phase in adolescents', *Sleep Medicine*, 8(6), 602–612. Available at: https://pubmed.ncbi.nlm.nih.gov/17383934/

19. National Institutes of Health (2020). 'Melatonin'. MedlinePlus. Available at: https://medlineplus.gov/druginfo/natural/940.html

20. Mindell, J. A. and Owens, J. A. (2015). *A Clinical Guide to Pediatric Sleep: Diagnosis and Management of Sleep Problems*. 3rd ed. Philadelphia: Wolters Kluwer.

21. American Academy of Sleep Medicine (n.d.) 'Confusional arousals'. Available at: https://sleepeducation.org/sleep-disorders/confusional-arousals

22. Mahowald, M. W. and Schenck, C. H. (2000). 'NREM sleep parasomnias', *Neurologic Clinics*, 18(4), 977–999. Available at: https://pubmed.ncbi.nlm.nih.gov/8923490/

23. Kirk, V. and Baughn, J. (2015). 'Sleepwalking', *UpToDate*. Available at: https://www.uptodate.com

24. Levin, R. and Nielsen, T. A. (2007). 'Disturbed dreaming, posttraumatic stress disorder, and affect distress: a review and neurocognitive model', *Psychological Bulletin*, 133(3), 482–528. Available at: https://pubmed.ncbi.nlm.nih.gov/17469988/

25. The Continuity Hypothesis, proposed by John Bowlby in 1953 in relation to dreams, suggests that our dreams are a continuation of

our waking life, helping us process emotions, solve problems and integrate new information. This understanding can be valuable in both therapeutic settings and personal self-reflection, providing a deeper insight into the connection between our daily experiences and our dreams.

26. Kirk, V., Baughn, J., D'Andrea, L., Friedman, N., Galion, A., Garetz, S., Hassan, F., Ishman, S. L., Jacobowitz, O., Katz, E. S., Mitchell, R. B. and Normand, S. (2020). 'Diagnosis and management of obstructive sleep apnea in childhood', *Pediatrics*, 145(1). Available at: https://doi.org/10.1542/peds.2019-2336

27. Sleep Foundation (n.d.). 'Delayed Sleep–Wake Phase Syndrome'. Available at: https://www.sleepfoundation.org

28. Roenneberg, T., Kuehnle, T., Pramstaller, P. P., Ricken, J., Havel, M., Guth, A. and Merrow, M. (2004). 'A marker for the end of adolescence', *Current Biology*, 14(24), R1038-R1039. Available at: https://pubmed.ncbi.nlm.nih.gov/15620633/

29. Narcolepsy UK (n.d.). 'About Narcolepsy'. Available at: https://www.narcolepsy.org.uk/about-narcolepsy/

30. Ibid.

31. Vilensky, J. A. and Gilman, S. (2006). 'Encephalitis lethargica: 100 years after the epidemic', *Brain*, 129(8), 2281–2282. Available at: https://pubmed.ncbi.nlm.nih.gov/28899018/

32. Leschziner, G. (2022). *The Neuroscience of Sleep and its Disorders*. Gresham College. Available at: https://www.youtube.com/watch?v=L-AFJDcoeZA

33. Postuma, R. B., Gagnon, J. F. and Montplaisir, J. Y. (2013). 'Rapid eye movement sleep behavior disorder as a biomarker for neurodegeneration', *The Lancet Neurology*, 12(5), 457–467. Available at: https://pubmed.ncbi.nlm.nih.gov/23058689/

34. Boeve, B. F., Silber, M. H. and Ferman, T. J. (2007). 'REM sleep behavior disorder in Parkinson's disease and dementia with Lewy bodies', *Journal of Geriatric Psychiatry and Neurology*, 20(1), 11–16. Available at: https://pubmed.ncbi.nlm.nih.gov/15312278/

35. Foley, D. J., Monjan, A. A., Brown, S. L., Simonsick, E. M., Wallace, R. B. and Blazer, D. G. (1995). 'Sleep complaints among elderly persons: an epidemiologic study of three communities', *Sleep*,

18(6), 425–432. Available at: https://pubmed.ncbi.nlm.nih.gov /7481413/

36. Ancoli-Israel, S. (2009). 'Sleep and its disorders in aging populations', *Sleep Medicine*, 10, S7–S11. Available at: https://pubmed.ncbi.nlm.nih .gov/19647483/

37. Ekerdt, D. J. (2010). 'Frontiers of research on work and retirement', *Journal of Gerontology: Social Sciences*, 65B (1), 69–80. Available at: https://pubmed.ncbi.nlm.nih.gov/20008480/

38. Kim, J. E. and Moen, P. (2002). 'Retirement transitions, gender, and psychological wellbeing: a life-course, ecological model', *The Journals of Gerontology: Series B*, 57(3), 212–222. Available at: https://pubmed .ncbi.nlm.nih.gov/11983732/

39. Crowley, K. (2011). 'Sleep and sleep disorders in older adults', *Neuropsychology Review*, 21(1), 41–53. Available at: https://pubmed .ncbi.nlm.nih.gov/21225347/

40. Vitiello, M. V. (2006). 'Sleep in normal ageing', *Sleep Medicine Clinics*, 1(2), 171–179. Available at: https://pubmed.ncbi.nlm.nih.gov /29412976/

41. Ibid.

42. Foley, D. J., Monjan, A. A., Brown, S. L., Simonsick, E. M., Wallace, R. B. and Blazer, D. G. (1995). 'Sleep complaints among elderly persons: an epidemiologic study of three communities', *Sleep*, 18(6), 425–432. Available at: https://pubmed.ncbi.nlm.nih .gov/7481413/

43. Ancoli-Israel, S. (2009). 'Sleep and its disorders in ageing populations', *Sleep Medicine*, 10, S7–S11. Available at: https:// pubmed.ncbi.nlm.nih.gov/19647483/

44. Canevelli, M., Valletta, M., Trebbastoni, A. et al. (2016). 'Sundowning in dementia: clinical relevance, pathophysiological determinants, and therapeutic approaches', *Frontiers in Medicine*, 3, 73. Available at: https://www.ncbi.nlm.nih.gov/pmc/articles/PMC5187352/

45. Dementia UK (n.d.). 'Sundowning'. Available at: https://www .dementiauk.org/information-and-support/health-advice /sundowning/

46. Ekerdt, D. J. (2010). 'Frontiers of research on work and retirement', *Journal of Gerontology: Social Sciences*, 65B(1), 69–80. Available at: https://pubmed.ncbi.nlm.nih.gov/20008480//

Appendix

1. Harvey, A. G. (2008). 'Sleep and circadian rhythms in bipolar disorder: seeking synchrony, harmony, and balance', *American Journal of Psychiatry*, 165(7), 820–9. Available at: https://doi: 10.1176/appi.ajp.2008.08010098

2. Foldvary-Schaefer, N. and Grigg-Damberger, M. (2006). 'Sleep and epilepsy: what we know, don't know, and need to know', *Journal of Clinical Neurophysiology*, 23(1), 4–20. doi.org/10.1097/01.wnp.0000206877.90232.cb